D0395612

FIRST AID

First Edition 1943 The Canadian Red Cross Society
© 18th Edition 1988—5th Printing

ISBN 0-920854-63-X

Acknowledgement

The Canadian Red Cross Society wishes to acknowledge the efforts of the many volunteers and staff involved in the development of this Manual. The growth and development of "First Aid" is a result of the work and dedication of hundreds of Canadians across the country. Although too numerous to mention, they know their efforts are fully recognized.

Credit also must be given to the League of Red Cross Societies and to our sister Society, the American Red Cross. Their guidance and resources have been invaluable. This manual is a reference for the Red Cross First Aid programme and it should not be considered a substitute for up-to-date training.

First Aid

"First Aid is the immediate assistance provided to a person in physical distress to maintain vital functions until qualified aid can be obtained".
-League of Red Cross Societies

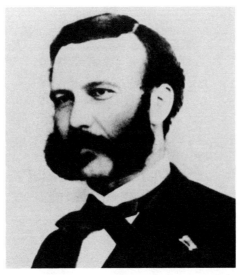

Henry Dunant.

PREFACE

On June 24, 1859 following the Battle of Solferino, 40,000 men lay wounded and dying. Into this field **Henry Dunant,** a Swiss banker, led volunteers he recruited to give First Aid care to the wounded. The injured were aided without prejudice; their wounds, not which side they fought on was the important issue, and so Red Cross was born. The purpose then and now is "the Improvement of health, the prevention of disease, and the mitigation of suffering throughout the world". One goal of the Canadian Red Cross is to provide the basic concepts of First Aid training to as many citizens as possible. By training people in the concepts of accident prevention and First Aid, we hope to significantly reduce the number of injuries sustained by Canadians.

First Aid

First Aid is the emergency measure required to:
* save lives
* prevent further injury
* ease pain and discomfort until qualified medical assistance is obtained.

Value of First Aid Training

* In an emergency, your First Aid knowledge and skill may mean the difference between life and death, temporary or permanent disability.
* The training provides guidelines for what to do and what not to do.
* By identifying your responsibilities and instructing you in how to take charge in an emergency, First Aid training promotes confidence.
* First aid training increases safety awareness through instruction in the causes, the effects and the prevention of accidents.

Legal Aspects of First Aid

The law expects you, the First Aider to be **cautious** when your actions affect others. You do not want to cause more harm than good while assisting a casualty.

There is no **general** legal duty to render assistance in an emergency. In specific cases such as motor vehicle accidents, however, any person **involved** in the accident is required to stop and give all possible assistance to the persons involved and report the accident to appropriate authorities.

The law does require that, once you begin giving emergency assistance to a casualty, **you must continue** until another qualified person is able to take over - preferably someone with medical training, unless you become too exhausted to continue or are at personal risk.

Section 216 cc of the Criminal Code provides that everyone who undertakes to administer surgical or medical treatment to another person or to do any other lawful acts that may endanger the life of another person is, except in cases of necessity, under a legal duty to have and to use reasonable knowledge, skill and care in so doing. Under Section 217 cc, everyone who undertakes to do an act is under a legal duty to do it if an omission to do the act is or may be dangerous to life.

What Should You Do?

1. Identify yourself to the casualty as a person trained in First Aid.
2. Ask the casualty if they want assistance, and only act if they wish your help.
3. If a young child requires emergency assistance and parental consent is not available, you can provide emergency aid.
4. If a casualty is unconscious, extend any emergency care necessary.

GIVE THE HELP THAT UNDER SIMILAR CIRCUMSTANCES YOU WOULD HOPE TO RECEIVE.

TABLE OF CONTENTS

Page

Chapter 1 Initial Assessment 2

Chapter 2 Airway Management 4

Chapter 3 Breathing 14

Chapter 4 Circulation 19

Chapter 5 Shock 24

Chapter 6 Poisons and Allergic Reactions 26

Chapter 7 How to Call for Emergency Medical Assistance 35

Chapter 8 Secondary Assessment 36

Chapter 9 Head and Spinal Injuries 38

Chapter 10 Bone and Joint Injuries 43

Chapter 11 Wounds 54

Chapter 12 Injuries Due to Heat or Cold 59

Chapter 13 Injuries to Specific Body Areas 66

Chapter 14 Medical Conditions 68

Chapter 15 Moving and Transportation 75

Chapter 16 Cardiopulmonary Resuscitation 81

Appendix First Aid Kit 91

Index 93

List of Figures 97

List of Tables 98

Chapter 1 — Initial Assessment

INITIAL ASSESSMENT

When an accident or sudden illness occurs, it is necessary to evaluate both the situation and the injuries. This evaluation is done in two stages:
1) Initial Assessment
2) Secondary Assessment

In an Initial Assessment, the First Aider deals with the examination and care for **LIFE-THREATENING PRIORITIES.**

A Secondary Assessment is carried out only **after** life-threatening priorities no longer exist. This assessment will identify further injuries which require attention, such as bone and joint injuries. Secondary assessment is explained in Chapter 8.

Initial Assessment:

Initial Assessment requires the First Aider to:
   a) approach the situation safely; and
   b) assess the casualty for life threatening priorities

A) APPROACH the situation

1. Environmental Safety

Proceed with caution so that you do not become the second casualty. **Do not assume** you know what happened. Look around. Ask bystanders, and the casualty if possible. The few seconds you take to determine the possible cause of the accident could save the casualty's life and your own. If further dangers like a fire or explosion are present, remove them if practical, or move the casualty to a safe location (see page 75 for environmental dangers).

2. Assessment of the Situation

If no one else is giving First Aid, be prepared to take charge.

You must determine, if possible, how the accident happened. By assessing the scene and asking bystanders you need to identify if there is a possible neck or spinal injury. This information will affect your assessment and immediate treatment of the casualty (see page 41 for care of spinal injuries).

B) ASSESS The casualty

Once you are certain it is safe to approach a casualty, you must quickly determine how to help. Your first priority is to ensure the Life Threatening Priorities are checked and treated. This involves the A,B,C's.

A. Airway —Is the airway clear?
             Is the casualty choking?
B. Breathing —Is the casualty breathing?
C. Circulation —Can you feel a pulse?
             Is the casualty bleeding severely?

By checking for these essential conditions, you will be able to identify which first aid techniques need to be applied immediately to maintain life.

Always follow up with a Call for Help. Get a bystander to call for an ambulance immediately and ensure your directions are followed (see page 35 for calling for help).

FIRST AID AND THE UNCONSCIOUS CASUALTY

If you find someone who has collapsed, you must first determine if they are unconscious.

Unconsciousness can be life threatening as the muscles relax, including the tongue, which could block the airway, causing breathing to stop. Follow these steps for the Unconscious Casualty.

FIRST AID FOR THE UNCONSCIOUS CASUALTY

STOP. How did the casualty get into this situation?

- Check environmental safety.
- Is a neck injury suspected? (see page 41).
- Check for unresponsiveness (shake the casualty's shoulder and ask "Are you okay"? If no response, assume the casualty is unconscious).
- Shout for help.
- If lying face down check for breathing without moving casualty.
- Turn over if not breathing. **NEVER move an unconscious casualty unnecessarily.**
- Open airway in appropriate manner, given circumstances. (see page 5 if neck/spinal injury suspected)
- Look, listen and feel for breathing. (3 to 5 seconds)
- Breathing may resume.
- If non-breathing, attempt rescue breathing. (See page 15-18)
- Check for pulse (see page 23). If pulse, resume rescue breathing. If no pulse begin CPR if trained (see page 69)
- Send someone to call an ambulance.

TABLE I.I INITIAL ASSESSMENT FLOW CHART

Activity	Must Do's
A. Approach the Situation	
1. Environmental Safety Assess safety of scene for a) yourself b) casualty	Danger removed or casualty removed from danger
2. Assessment of the Situation Assess cause of accident	QUICKLY - if possible determine how accident occured. Is a neck or Spinal injury suspected?
3. Instruct casualty to lie still (if conscious)	- Identify yourself as a First Aider - Offer reassurance
B. Assess the Casualty	
4. Assess ABC's - airway - breathing - circulation	- Check consciousness - Is the airway open? (see page 4-5) - Is the casualty breathing? (see page 15-18) - Is there a pulse? (see page 23) - Is there severe bleeding? (see page 20)
5. Send for help - Call ambulance	- Use bystanders (see page 35) if possible

3

Chapter 2 — Airway Management

There are two ways for a first aider to ensure the casualty has a clear airway.

1. Open the airway - using the appropriate technique given the circumstances
2. Remove an airway obstruction

1. OPENING THE AIRWAY

If you have determined that a casualty is unconscious (see page 3) you will want to ensure the airway is clear. If the unconscious casualty is lying on his back, the tongue (a muscle attached to the jaw) may fall to the back of the throat, blocking the airway and causing breathing to stop (see Figure 2.1). For this reason, the rescuer's first concern with an unconscious casualty should be the tongue, rather than foreign body obstruction.

It is essential to establish an open airway and restore breathing immediately. The casualty may begin breathing spontaneously after opening the airway; if not, rescue breathing may be necessary (see page 15-18).

NOTE: For reference throughout this text, an infant is birth - 1 year of age, a child is to 8 years of age and an adult is over 8 years of age.

OPENING THE AIRWAY - ADULT & CHILD (1-8 YEARS OLD)

The choice of method to open the airway is dictated by the circumstances surrounding the casualty. In the absence of complications, opening the airway, regardless of the technique used, is a matter of lifting the tongue away from the back of the throat. Special techniques are used for a suspected neck or spinal injury.

General Rules for the Uncomplicated Situation

When there is **no** reason to suspect a neck or spinal injury, the head tilt/chin lift method is most appropriate. One hand lifts the chin up while the other hand exerts pressure on the forehead, causing the head to tilt backwards. This pulls the tongue away from the back of the airway in most cases. (see Figure 2.2).

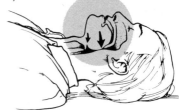

Figure 2.1
Obstruction of airway
caused by tongue.

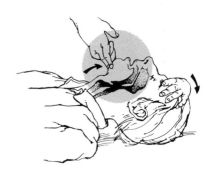

Figure 2.2
Opened Airway

General Rules for a Suspected Spinal Injury

1. If you did not see the casualty fall to the ground, assume a neck injury.

2. If the casualty fell with a great deal of force, assume a neck injury (for example, being thrown from a car or falling down a flight of stairs).

3. If the casualty has sustained an injury above the collarbone, assume a neck injury.

In such situations, a method known as the "jaw thrust" is the best method to minimize movement of the neck and still pull the tongue away from the back of the throat.

The head is held steady while the fingers are placed beneath the angle of the jaw which is then lifted up (See fig. 2.3). Since both hands are occupied, the First Aider must seal his mouth over the casualty's mouth so that his cheek blocks the casualty's nose. Do not hyper-extend the neck if a neck injury is suspected - simply lift the casualty's jaw.

If the airway remains blocked, the First Aider must tilt the head **slightly** back and try the jaw thrust again (see figure 2.4).

OPENING THE AIRWAY - INFANT (0-1 YEAR OLD)

Infant Airway Management. To open the airway of an infant, use the head tilt/chin lift method. Caution is necessary to avoid over-extending the neck since this may cause the airway to close, becoming pinched like a straw.

If attempts to ventilate meet with obstruction, carefully reposition the head and attempt to ventilate again. If still unsuccessful, assume airway is obstructed. Use obstructed airway procedures (see page 13).

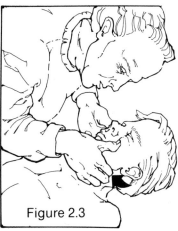

Figure 2.3

Jaw Thrust Maneouvre

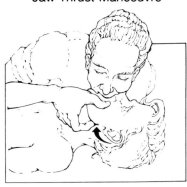

Figure 2.4
Jaw Thrust Maneouvre

2. Airway Obstructions

Both conscious and unconscious casualties may have an obstructed airway. In the conscious casualty, airway obstruction is most often caused by choking on a foreign object.

CHOKING

PREVENTION IS THE FIRST STEP IN FIRST AID FOR CHOKING

To prevent choking:
- cut food into small pieces
- chew food thoroughly
- avoid laughing, talking, walking or running with anything in your mouth
- ensure children keep objects out of their mouths

Be **EXTRA** careful while eating if:
- you wear dentures
- you have consumed alcohol

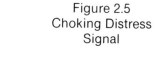

Figure 2.5
Choking Distress
Signal

Signs and Symptoms of Choking

A casualty may have a partial or complete airway obstruction. Learn to recognize the difference.

If Airway Obstruction is:	Signs & Symptoms Look for:	Action
Partial-Good Air Exchange	• Good air exchange • Casualty can speak or cough forcefully, breathe and speak or cough again • Often a high pitched sound on inhalation between coughs	• Do not interfere • Encourage casualty to continue coughing in an attempt to clear the airway • Go with the casualty if he/she leaves the room
Partial-Poor Air Exchange	• Poor air exchange • Casualty has a weak ineffectual cough • Unable to speak • Breathing may be accompanied by high pitched sound on inhalation • Lips and ear lobes may appear blue	• Treat as a complete airway obstruction (see page 8-13)
Complete-No Air Exchange	• No air exchange • Casualty is unable to speak or cough • May clutch throat in the choking distress signal (see figure 2.5) • May appear bluish in the face • Without action to remove obstruction unconsciousness will soon follow	• Treat as a complete airway obstruction (see page 8-13)

FIRST AID FOR CHOKING

Once you have determined that the casualty needs your help, prepare to perform the Heimlich Manoeuvre (abdominal thrusts).

WHAT TO DO

Ask the casualty "Are you choking?". Reassure the victim. Tell them you can help. If it is obvious that the casualty has not succeeded in inhaling air, prepare to perform the Heimlich Manoeuvre (abdominal thrusts). Speed is very important. Do not leave a choking casualty alone or let them go on their own to "cough it out".

THE HEIMLICH MANOEUVRE - CONSCIOUS CASUALTY

Stand behind the casualty and wrap your arms around the casualty's waist. Make a fist with one hand, and place the thumb side of this fist against the abdomen above the navel and well below the tip of the breastbone or xiphoid. Grasp the fist with the other hand, and press into the casualty's abdomen with quick, inward and upward thrusts. Continue the thrusts until the obstruction is successfully expelled or the casualty becomes unconscious (See Figure 2.6).

When **simulating** abdominal thrusts with a partner, encourage your "casualty" to open his mouth and say "AAH". This exhalation prevents increased internal pressure and/or damage to vital organs. Always demonstrate care and caution.

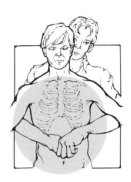

Figure 2.6
Heimlich
Manoeuvre
(Abdominal
Thrusts)

If you experience an airway obstruction yourself, you can perform the Heimlich Manoeuvre alone.

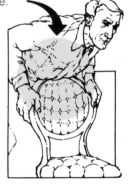

Figure 2.7
Self
administered
abdominal
thrusts

Techniques are similar to those for a conscious casualty. Make a fist with one hand and place the thumb side on the abdomen above the navel and below the tip of the breastbone. Grasp the fist with your other hand, and press inward and upward toward the diaphragm with a quick motion.

If this is not successful, press your upper abdomen quickly over any firm surface such as the back of a chair or side of a table. Several thrusts may be needed to clear the airway. (See Figure 2.7)

WHAT TO DO FOR A COMPLETE AIRWAY OBSTRUCTION CONSCIOUS ADULT AND CHILD

STEPS	RESCUE ACTIVITY	MUST DO'S
1	• Rescuer asks: "Are you choking?" • Reassure casualty - say, I can help" • Do not leave the casualty alone	• Rescuer must identify complete airway obstruction by asking if he/she is choking
2	• Heimlich Manoeuvre (6-10 Abdominal Thrusts)	• Stand behind casualty and encircle the waist • Locate correct hand position • Grasp one fist with the other hand (thumb side in) • Press fist into abdomen with upward-inward thrust of increasing force • Caution - Adjust the force of the thrust to the size of a child. Use less force for a smaller child
3	• Repeat manoeuvre until the object is expelled or the casualty becomes unconscious	• As above • Seek medical attention immediately • Care for shock (see page 24)

A CONSCIOUS CASUALTY (ADULT OR CHILD) BECOMES UNCONSCIOUS

4	• Assist the casualty to the floor • Shout for HELP • Send someone to call an ambulance	• Support the head and neck • Gently lay the casualty on the floor, face up.
5	• Foreign Body Check	• Tongue-jaw lift • Finger sweep (for adults) • Caution - Do not perform a blind finger sweep on a child or infant. in the the child's mouth. If you can see the object, remove it, taking care not to push it in any further.
6	• Attempt ventilation (airway is obstructed)	• Head tilt/chin lift • Seal mouth and nose • Give 2 slow breaths

7	• Heimlich Manoeuvre (6-10 Abdominal Thrusts) (See Figure 2.8)	• Straddle casualty's thighs • Place hands on the casualty's abdomen, above the navel and well below the xiphoid. • Press into abdomen with quick upward thrusts • Caution - Adjust the force of the thrust to the size of the casualty. Use less force for a smaller child.
8	• Continue with steps 5, 6 and 7	• Repeat sequence until successful • Seek medical attention • When the object is expelled be prepared to perform rescue breathing (see page 15) or CPR (see page 81) • Care for shock (see page 24)

Caution - If a casualty is pregnant or extremely obese, you may need to perform chest thrusts until the object is expelled or the casualty becomes unconscious.

Stand behind the casualty, with arms under their armpits at chest level. Grab one fist with the other hand and place the thumb side on the middle of the breastbone. Press the breastbone with quick backward thrusts. These are performed until the object is expelled or the casualty becomes unconscious. If the casualty becomes unconscious, place them flat on the back. Position yourself beside the casualty and continue chest-thrusts with hands placed on top of each other on the middle of the breastbone. Continue chest thrusts until the object is expelled or emergency medical help arrives.

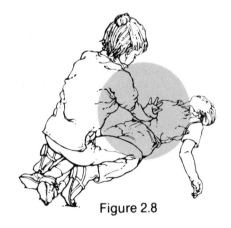

Figure 2.8

Heimlich Manoeuvre
(Unconscious Casualty)

WHAT TO DO FOR A COMPLETE AIRWAY OBSTRUCTION: UNCONSCIOUS ADULT OR CHILD (1-8 YEARS):

STEPS	RESCUE ACTIVITY	MUST DO'S
1	• Establish unresponsiveness • Call for help • Position the casualty • Open airway • Establish breathlessness	• Shake shoulder; ask "Are you O.K.?" • Shout for HELP • Turn if necessary (one continuous movement) • Look, listen and feel
2	• Attempt ventilation (airway is obstructed)	• Head tilt/chin lift • Seal mouth and nose
3	• Reposition head • Re-attempt ventilation (airway remains blocked) • Call an ambulance	• Refer to Step 2
4	• Heimlich Manoeuvre (6-10 Abdominal Thrusts) (See Figure 2.8)	• Straddle casualty's thighs • Place hands on casualty's abdomen above the navel and well below the xiphoid or the tip of the breastbone. • Press into abdomen with quick, upward thrusts • Caution - adjust the force of the thrust to the size of the casualty. Use less force for a smaller child.
5	• Foreign Body Check	• Tongue-jaw lift • Finger sweep • Caution - Do not perform a blind finger sweep for children or infants. If you can see the object remove it, taking care not to push it in any further
6	• Attempt ventilation	• Head tilt/chin lift • Seal mouth and nose
7	• Continue with steps 4, 5 and 6	• As above • Repeat sequence until successful • Seek medical attention • When object is expelled, be prepared to perform rescue breathing (see page 15) or CPR (see page 81) • Care for shock (see page 24)

WHAT TO DO FOR A COMPLETE AIRWAY OBSTRUCTION
CONSCIOUS INFANT (BIRTH - 1 YEAR)

STEPS	RESCUE ACTIVITY	MUST DO'S
1	• Observe difficulty in breathing • Shout for help • Position the infant	• Identify complete airway obstruction • Turn infant face down on your arm with the head lower lower than the body • Support the head and neck
2	• Deliver 4 back blows	• Use the heel of your hand to deliver 4 sharp back blows between the shoulder blades
3	• Deliver 4 chest thrusts	• Turn the infant over, face up in your lap with head lower than the body, support the head • Place 3 fingers on the breast bone between the infant's nipples • Lift the index finger • Use 2 fingers for 4 chest thrusts (compress 1.3-2.5cm (½" to 1")
4	• Continue with steps 2 & 3	• As above • Repeat sequence until successful • Seek medical attention • Care for Shock (see page 24)

A CONSCIOUS INFANT BECOMES UNCONSCIOUS

STEPS	RESCUE ACTIVITY	MUST DO'S
5	• Send someone to call an ambulance • Position the infant • Ensure help is coming	• Place infant onto its back • Support the head and neck
6	• Foreign Body Check • No blind finger sweeps	• Grasp the tongue and lower jaw. Look into the mouth. If you can see the object, remove it, taking care not to push it in further
7	• Attempt ventilation (if aiway is still obstructed)	• If you cannot remove the object, head tilt/chin lift • Avoid over-extension of the infant's neck as this may close the airway • Seal mouth and nose • Attempt to deliver 2 small puffs of air

11

8	• Deliver 4 back blows & 4 chest thrusts	• Repeat steps 2 & 3
9	• Foreign Body Check	• Repeat step 6
10	• Continue with steps 7-9	• Repeat until successful • When the object is expelled be prepared to perform rescue breathing (see page 17) or CPR (see page 81) • Seek medical attention • Care for Shock (see page 24)

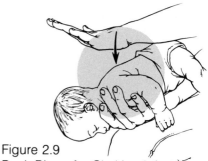

Figure 2.9
Back Blows for Choking Infant

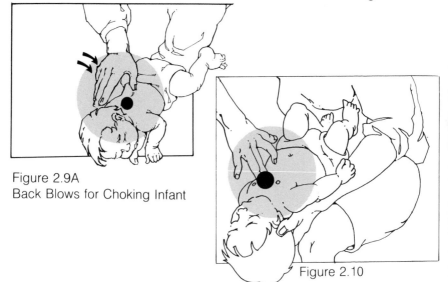

Figure 2.9A
Back Blows for Choking Infant

Figure 2.10
Chest Thrusts for Choking Infant

COMPLETE AIRWAY OBSTRUCTION
UNCONSCIOUS INFANT

STEPS	RESCUE ACTIVITY	MUST DO'S
1	• Establish unresponsiveness • Shout for help • Open the airway • Establish breathlessness	• Tap the infant & call his name • If no response, shout for help • Turn if necessary • Look, listen and feel • Caution - Do not over-extend the neck
2	• Attempt ventilation	• Seal mouth and nose • Deliver 2 small puffs of air
3	• Reattempt ventilation (if airway is still obstructed)	• Reposition infant's head • Send someone to call an ambulance
4	• Deliver 4 back blows & 4 chest thrusts	• See conscious choking infant, (page 11) steps 2 & 3 • Position infant face down on your arm with the head lower than the trunk. Support the head & neck
5	• Foreign Body Check • No blind finger sweeps	• Grasp the tongue and lower jaw. Look into the mouth. If you can see the object remove it, taking care not to push it in further
6	• Attempt ventilation	• Head tilt/chin lift • Seal mouth and nose • Deliver 2 small puffs of air
7	• Continue with steps 4-6	• Repeat until successful • When object is expelled, be prepared to perform rescue breathing (see page 17) or CPR (see page 81) • Seek medical attention • Care for shock (see page 24)

Chapter 3 — Breathing

Breathing is an automatic action. It continues rhythmically, without voluntary effort. Controlled by our brain's respiratory centre, our breathing involves many structures, but mainly the mouth and nose, the windpipe, lungs, diaphragm and chest muscles. LIFE DEPENDS ON AN ADEQUATE SUPPLY OF OXYGEN REACHING THE BRAIN.

When there is interference with the quantity or quality of this oxygen, there is danger of suffocation and death. **Brain damage may begin to occur if a casualty is without oxygen for more than 4-6 minutes.**

CAUSES: LOSS OF BREATHING

1. **Obstruction of the air passage. May be caused by:**
   a) tongue
   b) a foreign body
   c) drowning
   d) asphyxiation (strangulation, smothering)

2. **Air lacking enough oxygen or containing poisonous gases:**
   a) domestic gases, engine exhaust fumes, dense smoke (carbon monoxide is the deadly gas in many cases).
   b) industrial gases such as ammonia gas, sulphur dioxide, or hydrogen sulfide.

3. **Interruption of the respiratory centre in the brain:**
   a) with electric shock

b) with poisons (e.g. a drug overdose and some gases)
c) through diseases
d) from head injuries
e) from spinal injuries

SIGNS: LOSS OF BREATHING
- No chest movement, or breathing sounds.
- Discolouration of face, lips, fingernails.
- Collapse and loss of consciousness.

First Aid for Loss of Breathing
The first aid for any casualty, adult, child or infant, who is not breathing is to begin RESCUE BREATHING. The most effective methods are mouth-to-mouth and mouth-to-nose. **For Rescue Breathing - Adult and Child see page 15. For Rescue Breathing - Infant see page 17. Mouth-to-nose - see page 18.**

RESCUE BREATHING - ADULT AND CHILD (1 to 8 years old)

STEPS	ACTIVITY	MUST DO'S
1	• Establish unresponsiveness • Shout for help • Position the casualty • Open airway	• Shake casualty's shoulder and ask "Are you O.K.?" • Send some for an ambulance • Turn if necessary • Head tilt/chin lift • If a neck or head injury is suspected, do a jaw thrust (see page 5)
2	• Establish breathlessness • Look, listen & feel for 6-10 seconds	• Kneel beside the casualty • Maintain open airway • Ear over mouth & nose, observe chest
3	• Breathing - Yes? - No?	• Maintain open airway, proceed to pulse check (see step 6) • Pinch nostrils closed with thumb and forefinger • Seal your mouth tightly around the casualty's mouth • Proceed to step 4
4	• 2 slow breaths • Caution - Use less force and volume on a child than for an adult. If the chest rises, the casualty is receiving air	• Give 2 slow breaths of air • Allow deflation between breaths • Remove your mouth • Release the nostrils • Listen for air escaping and watch for chest movement • If chest movement occurs, begin step 6
5	• If no chest movement	• Readjust head tilt • Attempt ventilation • If chest still does not move, perform obstructed airway techniques (see page 10)

6	• Check Pulse	• If airway is clear and casualty is breathing or chest movement occurs with rescue breathing, check for a pulse (see page 23)
		• If pulse, continue rescue breathing (step 7)
		• If no pulse, begin CPR if trained (see page 81)
		• Call an ambulance
7	• Continue Rescue Breathing Cycle	• Open airway, pinch nostrils, seal mouth
		• Adult - give one full breath every 5 seconds
		• Child - give one full breath every 4 seconds, adjust to size of child
		• Continue until successful, or an ambulance arrives
8	• If casualty vomits	• Roll as a unit on side
		• Clean out the mouth
		• Resume Rescue Breathing (step 7)
9	• Care for shock	• See page 24
		• Ensure an ambulance is coming

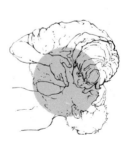

Fig. 3.1
Mouth-to-Mouth Seal
Adult and Child

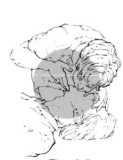

Fig. 3.3
Mouth-to-Mouth and Nose
Seal — Adult and Infant

Fig. 3.2
Mouth-to-Mouth Technique
Adult and Adult

RESCUE BREATHING — INFANT (BIRTH – 1 YEAR)

STEPS	RESCUE ACTIVITY	MUST DO'S
1	• Establish unreponsiveness • Shout for help • Position the infant • Open the airway • For an infant be careful not to over-extend the neck	• Tap infant and call their name • Shout for help • Turn if necessary • Head tilt/chin lift • If a head or neck injury is suspected, gently lift the lower neck. Tilt the head **only** if you cannot inflate the chest
2	• Establish breathlessness • Look, listen & feel for 3-5 seconds	• Place your cheek over the infant's mouth and nose • Listen and feel for air, watch for chest movement
3	• Breathing — Yes? No?	• Maintain open airway • Proceed to pulse check (step 6) • Seal your mouth over the infant's mouth and nose. Continue to step 4
4	• Give 2 slow puffs of air • Caution - Use much less force and volume for an infant that for a child or adult • If the chest rises, you are putting in enough air	• Deliver 2 small slow puffs of air • Take your mouth away each time and allow the lungs to deflate • If chest movement, proceed to pulse check (step 6)
5	• If no chest movement	• Readjust head tilt (step 1) • Attempt 2 more puffs • If still unsuccessful, perform obstructed airway techniques (see page 13)
6	• Check pulse	• Check the brachial pulse on the infant (see page 23) • If pulse, continue rescue breathing (step 7) • If no pulse, begin CPR if trained (see page 81) • Call an ambulance

7	Continue Rescue Breathing cycle	• Open airway, seal mouth and nose • Give one small puff of air every 3 seconds • Continue until successful or an ambulance arrives
8	If infant vomits	• Roll as a unit onto side • Clean out the mouth • Resume rescue breathing (step 7)
9	Care for shock	• see page 24

Ensure a casualty who begins breathing with your aid is transferred to medical facilities immediately.

MOUTH TO NOSE BREATHING

The mouth-to-nose method of Rescue Breathing may be used if the rescuer cannot make a seal for the mouth-to-mouth method because of injuries to the casualty's mouth, jaw fractures, lack of dentures or the casualty's position. Mouth-to-nose Rescue Breathing is similar to mouth-to-mouth, but the rescuer seals the casualty's mouth with one hand and inflates the lungs by blowing through the casualty's nose. (see Figure 3.4). After inflating the lungs, the mouth may have to be opened to allow for exhalation.

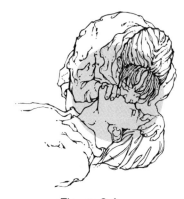

Figure 3.4
Mouth to Nose Technique

MOUTH TO STOMA

Mouth-to-stoma (neck opening). For a casualty who breathes through an opening in the neck, seal the mouth and nose. Then follow the remaining steps of mouth-to-mouth, by breathing into the stoma (see Figure 3.5).

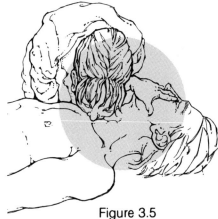

Figure 3.5
Mouth to Stoma Technique

Chapter 4 — Circulation

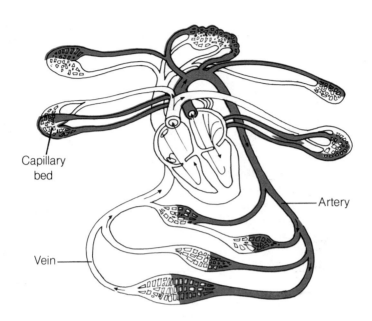

Capillary bed

Artery

Vein

Figure 4.1: Schematic circulatory system

BLEEDING

Our normal blood circulation system involves the heart and blood vessels. (see Figure 4.1). It is a continuous system for transporting blood from the heart to all parts of the body and back again. The major types of blood vessels in the circulatory system are called arteries, veins and capillaries.

Arteries are blood vessels which carry blood from the heart to all parts of the body; they are under high pressure. If severed, the bleeding will be profuse and will spurt in rhythm with the heart beat.

If a major artery is involved, this is a life threatening situation and must be controlled immediately.

Veins are blood vessels which carry blood from all parts of the body back to the heart; they are under relatively low pressure. Venous bleeding will tend to flow continuously.

Capillaries are microscopic vessels located in all tissues of the body. They are thin-walled. In these vessels the exchange of oxygen, nutrients and wastes occurs between the blood and body tissues.

EXTERNAL BLEEDING

- External bleeding (visible) occurs most often through a break in the skin.

FIRST AID FOR EXTERNAL BLEEDING

- **Quickly apply direct pressure** to the bleeding area with the cleanest material available. The hand must be used if nothing else is immediately available (see Figure 4.2 and 4.3).
- Have the casualty lie down and keep still.
- Apply a pressure bandage, using a folded clean dressing held firmly in place with bandages or a suitable substitute.
- **Elevate** the injured area if practical, unless fracture is suspected.
- Care for shock (see page 24)
- Reassure the casualty and cover over and under to maintain body warmth.
- No food or fluids should be given to the casualty.
- Check the casualty's breathing.
- Check colour and sensation of extremity to ensure pressure bandage is not tied too tightly.
- Seek medical attention for the injury.

NEVER REMOVE A PRESSURE BANDAGE. If the first bandage becomes blood soaked add another pressure bandage over the first.

Severe bleeding from the neck must be controlled with dressings and hand pressure, being careful not to obstruct the airway.

CAUTION: DO NOT PRESS ON BOTH SIDES OF THE THROAT AT ONCE. **DO NOT** MAINTAIN PRESSURE BY WRAPPING A PRESSURE BANDAGE AROUND A PERSON'S THROAT.

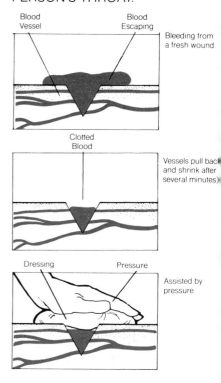

Blood Vessel

Blood Escaping

Bleeding from a fresh wound.

Clotted Blood

Vessels pull back and shrink after several minutes.

Dressing

Pressure

Assisted by pressure

Figure 4.2: Control of bleeding

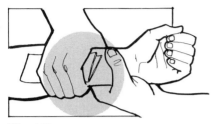

Direct Pressure

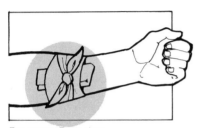

Pressure Dressing

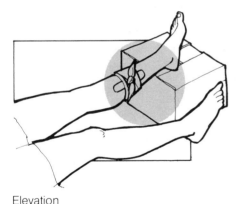

Elevation

Figure 4.3: First aid for severe bleeding

INTERNAL BLEEDING:

There are two types of internal bleeding, concealed and visible.

- **CONCEALED** – The bleeding is not visible. The blood passes into a body cavity which has no natural opening, such as the skull, chest or abdomen.
- **VISIBLE** – The blood comes to the outside through natural openings such as the nose, mouth or rectum.

Signs and Symptoms of Internal Bleeding

- pale skin colour
- cool, clammy skin
- sweating
- severe thirst
- increased sensitivity or pain over the injured site
- air hunger (yawning or gasping)
- a fainting feeling

FIRST AID FOR INTERNAL BLEEDING

- Reassure the casualty.
- Keep the casualty in a semi-prone position. (see page 25)
- Care for shock (see page 24)

- Maintain body temperature by providing light covering over and under for the casualty.
- No fluids are to be administered.
- Watch for changes (see Secondary Assessment page 36)
- Seek medical attention immediately.

"Sucking" Wound of the Chest Wall

A "sucking" chest-wound results from a puncture of the chest wall. It allows air to flow in and out of the chest cavity with each breath. This injury requires immediate attention. (see Figure 4.4)

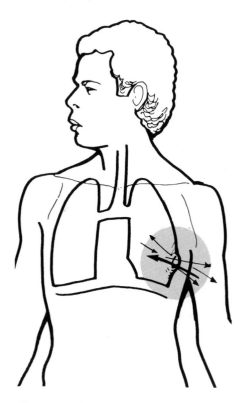

Figure 4.4: Schematic: Sucking chest wound

FIRST AID FOR A "SUCKING" WOUND OF THE CHEST WALL

- Stop the "sucking" by making a seal over the opening, **preferably following expiration.** Use any means at your disposal to make the seal: a piece of plastic film, adhesive strapping or even your own hand. Leave one edge of the seal free to allow for air to escape.
- Place the casualty in a semi-prone position, **injured side down** to allow for drainage.
- Make the casualty as comfortable as possible and care for shock. (see page 24)
- Check for any changes in condition. (see page 36)
- Seek medical attention for the injury.

IMPALED OBJECTS

An object which pierces a casualty's body and remains embedded is an impaled object and should not be removed.

First Aid for Impaled Objects:

- Do not remove the object
- Stabilize the object with bulky dressings or a ring bandage around it (see page 23)
- Secure the stabilizing items with pressure bandages
- Cover the object lightly (if possible)
- Care for shock (see page 24)
- Check for any changes in condition (see page 36)
- Seek medical attention for the injury

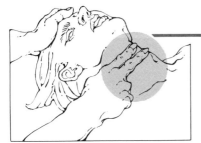

Fig. 4.6 Pulse Check (Landmark)

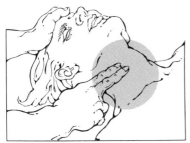

Fig. 4.7 Pulse Check (Location)

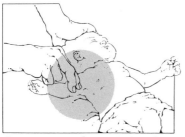

Fig. 4.8 Pulse Check (Infant Brachial)

PULSE CHECK

Checking the pulse of a casualty is done after breathing is assessed and rescue breathing if necessary is started. The absence of a pulse means CPR must be started immediately (see page 69). Use your fingers only, not your thumb, since you may mistake your pulse for that of the casualty.

Pulse Check – Adult & Child

Always take the pulse on the side closest to you.

1. Place your fingertips on the side of the casualty's windpipe, halfway between the casualty's chin and collarbone. Do not reach across the windpipe.
2. Press gently into the soft area beside the windpipe. Feel for the pulse for 5-10 seconds.

Pulse Check – Infant (Brachial pulse)

1. Place two fingertips close to the bone inside the infant's arm.
2. Press gently. Feel for the pulse for 5-10 seconds.

Figure 4.5 First Aid for Impaled Objects

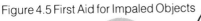

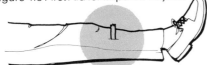

• Do not remove embedded object

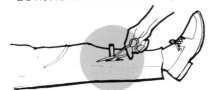

• Cut clothing away from injured site

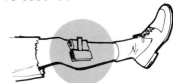

• Stabilize object with bulky dressings or a ring bandage

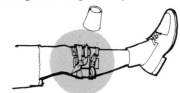

• Cover lightly

Chapter 5 — Shock

Shock is a condition in which the circulation of blood is inadequate to meet the oxygen needs of the body's vital tissues (i.e. brain, heart, lungs). This leads to a lack of oxygen to cells, cell death and possible death of the casualty.

Signs and Symptoms of Shock

Early:

- pale
- cold, clammy skin
- weakness
- increased rate of breathing
- anxiety
- severe thirst
- vomiting
- confusion
- restlessness

Late:

- no interest and unresponsive
- sunken, vacant eyes
- possible lapse into unconsciousness

FIRST AID FOR SHOCK
(see Figure 5.1)

- Reassure the casualty. See that the casualty lies down.
- Cover the casualty to maintain body temperature (over and under).
- Elevate the casualty's feet if head, neck or spinal injury is not suspected and there is no fracture to the lower body.
- A casualty who is unconscious should be placed in a semi-prone or recovery position (see page 25) to maintain airway and allow for drainage of fluids.
- Seek medical attention for the casualty.
- Observe and note any changes in the casualty's condition (see page 36).
- Do not give the casualty any fluids or food.

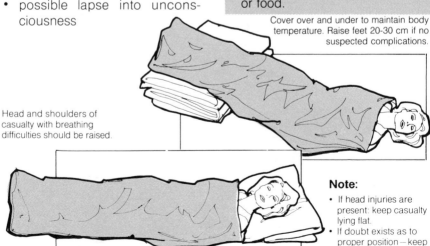

Cover over and under to maintain body temperature. Raise feet 20-30 cm if no suspected complications.

Head and shoulders of casualty with breathing difficulties should be raised.

Note:
- If head injuries are present: keep casualty lying flat.
- If doubt exists as to proper position — keep lying flat.

Figure 5.1: First aid for shock

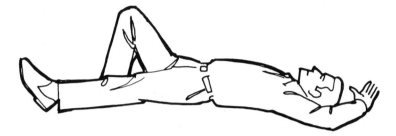

Raise casualty's closest arm above the head. Prepare to roll the casualty towards you.

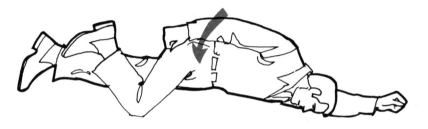

Gently roll as a unit. Guard the head as you roll the casualty.

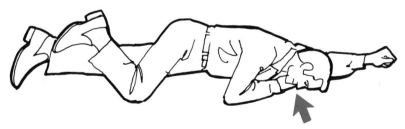

Tilt head to maintain airway. Tuck nearest hand under cheek to help maintain head tilt.

Figure 5.2: Semi-prone or Recovery Position

(for spontaneously breathing unconscious casualty).

Chapter 6 — Poisons And Allergic Reactions

A poison is any liquid, solid or gas which is harmful when introduced to the body. (see Tables 6.1, 6.2)

PREVENTION IS THE FIRST STEP IN FIRST AID FOR POISONING.

- **All** medicines should be placed in a locked cabinet preferably out of reach of children. **Remember that a safe dose of medicine for an adult may be a poisonous dose for a child.**
- All medicine bottles and boxes should be carefully labelled.
- Any unlabelled or old medicine should be destroyed by flushing it down the toilet.
- Medicine should never be taken in the dark, nor at any time when the label on the bottle cannot be read clearly. All medicine cabinets should have proper lighting.
- Labels should be read three times when the medicine is taken or given:

  First, when the container is selected.

  Second, when the dose is measured.

  Third, when the container is returned to the medicine cabinet.
- Remember, just because the recommended dosage is good — double the dosage is **not** better.
- Prescription medicine should only be taken by the person for whom it was prescribed.
- **Never** use containers such as beverage bottles to store toxic liquids, since they can be mistaken for other substances by a thirsty child or adult.
- Don't call medicines ''candy''.
- Bacteria rapidly produce poisons in unrefrigerated foods containing milk, cream, eggs, meat, fish or fowl. Strict cleanliness must be ensured when storing and handling food. Old refrigerated foods should be destroyed. Fruits and vegetables should be washed thoroughly to remove toxic sprays and dirt. Wash your hands well **before** and **after** handling food.
- Many plants, berries and seeds are poisonous. Use only those known to be safe.
- Do not run your car's engine in a closed garage or while you are parked.
- Do not use aerosol sprays in confined areas.
- Avoid contact with plants or chemicals which cause irritating reactions.

FIRST AID FOR POISONING

Poisons are classified by the way they enter the body.

a. INGESTED   SWALLOWED

b. INHALED   BREATHED IN BY NOSE OR MOUTH

c. INJECTED   THROUGH THE SKIN TO THE BLOOD STREAM

d. CONTACT   THROUGH TOUCHING THE SKIN OR EYES

FIRST AID FOR INGESTED POISONS

If the casualty is unconscious or semi-conscious, care for as an unconscious casualty and call for the ambulance.

Classification	First Aid Steps
(see Table 6.1 for examples) 1. Drugs and Medicines	-Give nothing by mouth. -Call Poison Centre or emergency medical facility for assistance.
2. Household Products or Chemicals (e.g. solvents, cleaning agents etc)	-Call Poison Centre or emergency medical facility for advice about whether/or not to induce vomiting. -If conscious, give water.
3. Unknown Agent	-Give nothing by mouth. -Call Poison Centre or emergency medical facility for assistance.

NOTE: IF POISON CAME FROM A CONTAINER, KEEP THE CONTAINER FOR USE BY POISON CENTRE. IF APPLICABLE, A SAMPLE OF VOMITUS SHOULD ALSO ACCOMPANY THE CASUALTY TO THE HOSPITAL.

NOTE: ALWAYS KEEP ON HANDS AT HOME A 30 cc (ONE OUNCE) BOTTLE OF SYRUP OF IPECAC FOR EACH CHILD IN THE HOME. USE ONLY ON THE ADVICE OF POISON CENTRE, OR EMERGENCY DEPARTMENT.

TABLE 6.1:

SOME POTENTIALLY DANGEROUS HOUSEHOLD POISONS

CLEANING BLEACHING AGENTS

Metal cleaners and polishes	Detergents
Ethylene glycol (anti-freeze)	Dry cleaning fluids
Lighter fluid	Benzene
Carbon tetrachloride	Ammonia
Copper and brass cleaner	Turpentine
Cleaning fluids	Alcohol
Gun cleaners	Kerosene
Methyl alcohol	Naphtha (i.e. fuel for camping stoves, lanterns, etc.)
Bleach	
Petroleum distillates	Window washing fluid
Drain cleaners	Typewriter cleaner
Aerosols	Oven cleaner
Bathroom bowl cleaner	

DRUGS AND MEDICINES

Narcotics	Antiseptics
Vitamins	A.S.A. (Aspirin)
Iron medicines	Pain killers
Clinitest tablets	Rubbing alcohol
Corn and wart remover	Iodine
Tranquilizers	Birth control pills
Laxatives	Children's fever drops
Cough syrup	Any prescription or over the counter (drugstore) medication

Note: Most of the items in this category are only poisonous when taken orally by accident or in excess.

SOLVENTS

Paint remover

Grease spot remover

Nail polish remover

Carbon tetrachloride

Methyl alcohol

Turpentine

Wax remover

Lacquer remover

Paint thinner

Kerosene

Petroleum products

Lighter fluid

POLISHES AND WAXES

Nail polish

Car wax

Silver polish

Mineral oil

Naptha

Furniture wax/polish

Kerosene

Pine oil

Turpentine

Paint

COSMETIC PREPARATIONS

Nail polish remover

Eye make-up

Corn and wart remover

Shaving lotions/creams

Suntan lotions

Cuticle removers

Permanent-wave solution

Hair dyes/tints

Neutralizers

Skin preparations

Hair sprays

Dandruff shampoo

Nail polish

After shave lotion

Hair lotions

Resins

Cologne

Bubble bath

Hair remover

Lacquers

Plasticizers

Perfume

Source: Heath and Welfare Canada

TABLE 6.2:

Common Poisonous Plants

PLANT	TOXIC PART	SYMPTOMS
Hyacinth Narcissus Daffodil	Bulbs	Nausea, vomiting, diarrhea. May be fatal.
Oleander	Leaves, Branches	Extremely poisonous. Affect heart, produce upset and have caused death.
Poinsettia	Sap	Can be irritating to skin and mucous membranes. Wash skin with soap and water. If ingested, vomiting and diarrhea may occur, and medical attention should be sought.
Dieffenbachia Elephant Ear	All parts	Intense burning and irritation of the mouth and tongue. Death can occur if base of the tongue swells enough to block the air passage.
Rosary pea Castor bean	Seeds	Fatal. A single rosary pea seed has caused death. One or two castor bean seeds are near the lethal dose for adults.
Mistletoe	Berries	Fatal. Both children and adults have died from the berries.
FLOWER GARDEN PLANTS		
Larkspur	Young plant, Seeds	Digestive upset, nervous excitement, depression. May be fatal.
Autumn crocus, Star-of- Bethlehem	Bulbs	Vomiting and nervous excitement.
Lily-of-the- valley	Leaves, Flowers	Irregular heart beat and pulse, usually accompanied by digestive upset and mental concussion.
Iris	Underground stems	Severe, but not usually serious, digestive upset.
Foxglove	Leaves	One of the sources of the drug digitalis, used to stimulate the heart. In large amounts, the active principles cause dangerously irregular heartbeat and pulse, usually digestive upset and mental confusion. May be fatal.

TABLE 6.2 (CONT.)

Bleeding heart (Dutchman's Breeches)	Foliage, Roots	May be poisonous in large amounts. Has proven fatal to cattle.

VEGETABLE GARDEN PLANTS

Rhubarb	Leaf blade	Fatal. Large amounts of raw or cooked leaves can cause convulsions, coma, followed rapidly by death.

ORNAMENTAL PLANTS

Daphne	Berries	Fatal. A few berries can kill a child.
Wisteria	Seeds pods	Mild to severe digestive upset. Many children are poisoned by this plant.
Golden chain	Bean-like capsules in which the seeds are suspended	Severe poisoning. Excitement, staggering, convulsions and coma. May be fatal.
Laurels, Rhododendron, Azaleas	All parts	Fatal. Produce nausea and vomiting, depression, difficult breathing, prostration and coma.
Jessamine	Berries	Fatal. Digestive disturbance and nervous symptoms.
Lantana Camara (Red Sage)	Green berries	Fatal. Affects lungs, kidneys, heart and nervous system. Grows in the U.S. and in moderate climates.
Yew	Berries, Foliage	Fatal. Foliage more toxic than berries. Death is usually sudden without warning signs.

TREES AND SHRUBS

Wild and cultivated cherries	Twigs Foliage	Fatal. Contains a compound that releases cyanide when eaten. Gasping, excitement, and prostration are common signs that often appear within minutes.
Oaks	Foliage, Acorns	Affects kidneys gradually, symptoms appear only after several days or weeks. Takes a large amount for poisoning. Children should not be allowed to chew on acorns.

TABLE 6.2 (CONT.)

Elderberry	All parts, especially roots	Children have been poisoned by using pieces of the pithy stems for blowguns. Nausea and digestive upset.
Black locust	Bark, spouts, foliage	Children have suffered nausea, weakness and depression after chewing the bark and seeds.
PLANTS IN WOODED AREAS		
Jack-in-the-pulpit	All parts, especially roots	Like dumb cane, contains needle-like crystals of calcium oxalate that cause intense irritation and burning of the mouth and tongue.
Moonseed	Berries	Resemble wild grapes, but contain only a single seed (wild grapes contain several small seeds). May be fatal.
Mayapple	Apple, foliage, roots	Contains at least 15 active toxic principles, primarily in the roots. Children often eat the apple with no ill effects, but several apples may cause diarrhea.
PLANTS IN FIELDS		
Buttercups	All parts	Irritant juices may severely injure the digestive system.
Nightshade	All parts, especially the unripe berry	Fatal. Intense digestive and nervous systems disturbances.
Poison hemlock	All parts	Fatal. Resembles a large wild carrot. Used in ancient Greece to kill condemned prisoners.
Jimson weed (thorn apple)	All parts	Abnormal thirst, distorted sight, delirium, incoherence and coma. Common cause of poisoning. Has proved fatal.

FIRST AID FOR INHALED POISONS

- Ensure your own safety first.
- Get casualty to fresh air immediately.
- If unconscious, see page 75 for instructions on how to move the casualty.
- Avoid breathing fumes.
- Start rescue breathing if casualty's breathing has stopped (see page 15-18) and CPR (see page 81) if their heart has stopped.
- Call Poison Centre for assistance.
- Care for Shock (see page 24).

FIRST AID FOR INJECTED POISONS

(see pages 33-34 on Insect Stings and Bites)

FIRST AID FOR CONTACT POISONS

- Remove contaminated clothing while flooding the skin with water for at least 10 minutes.
- Call Poison Centre for assistance

NOTE: FOR POISONS IN CONTACT WITH THE EYES

- Flood with lukewarm water poured from 5-10 cm (2-4 inches) above the injured eye.
- Avoid washing contaminants into uninjured eye.
- Continue flooding for 10-15 minutes.
- Have casualty blink constantly -DO NOT FORCE EYELID OPEN.

ALLERGIC REACTIONS

These are reactions by a person overly sensitive to some foreign substances, often certain foods, drugs, insect venom, pollen, etc.

SIGNS AND SYMPTOMS OF ALLERGIC REACTIONS

- Weakness.
- Pale skin colour.
- Difficulty in breathing on exhalation.
- Puffiness or swelling of tissues, especially near the eyes or throat.
- Itchy skin; sometimes a rash will occur also.
- With some allergic reactions the person may collapse if not cared for immediately.

FIRST AID FOR ALLERGIC REACTIONS

- Look for medical identification (see page 37).
- If the casualty stops breathing give Rescue Breathing (see page 15-18) and CPR (see page 81) if their heart stops.
- Care for shock (see page 24).
- Seek immediate medical attention for the allergy.

BEE AND WASP STINGS (Allergic reaction).

SIGNS AND SYMPTOMS OF BEE AND WASP STINGS

- Pain, redness and swelling at the site of sting, followed in some cases by an extreme allergic reaction involving difficulty in breathing, loss of consciousness.

FIRST AID FOR BEE AND WASP STINGS

- Check for medical identification.
- Ask the casualty if they carry a sting kit.
- Apply a cold compress.
- Make sure a casualty who is having difficulty breathing has an open airway. If the casualty stops breathing give Rescue Breathing (see page 15-18) and CPR (see page 81) if their heart stops.
- Seek medical attention **immediately** for the casualty if signs of an allergic reaction are apparent. (see page 33).
- Care for shock (see page 24).

If it is determined that the casualty is not prone to allergic reactions, the First Aider should:

- remove the stinger by gently scraping it off the skin. **DO NOT SQUEEZE THE STINGER** by using tweezers or forceps. This could cause the stinger to inject more poison.

ALCOHOL AND DRUG ABUSE

Any chemical taken frequently in large amounts, that affects the normal functioning of the body or mind, is a case of drug abuse.

PREVENTION IS THE FIRST STEP IN FIRST AID FOR ALCOHOL AND DRUG ABUSE.

For information on the prevention of alcohol and drug abuse, please contact your local office which deals with substance abuse or addiction.

SIGNS AND SYMPTOMS OF DRUG ABUSE

(in increasing order of severity)

- Restlessness, muscle twitching
- Reddened, glazed or blank staring eyes.
- Changes in mood and personality
- Delusions and hallucinations may occur
- Violence, irrational behaviour may follow
- Seizure or Unconsciousness.

FIRST AID FOR DRUG ABUSE

- Make sure the casualty has an open airway.
- Give Rescue Breathing if the casualty is unconscious and not breathing (see page 15-18) and CPR (see page 81) if their heart stops.
- Care for shock (see page 24)
- Call Poison Centre for assistance.
- If possible, identify the drug and report the type when informing poison centre.
- If the casualty is violent, stay clear and call the police.
- A casualty who is conscious, but sluggish and uninterested should be kept moving and talking if possible.
- Seek medical attention as indicated in cases of drug abuse.
- Send pills, bottles, labels and sample of vomitus with casualty to hospital.

Chapter 7 — How to Call For Emergency Medical Assistance

BEFORE CALLING FOR HELP

- Check emergency numbers for ambulance, police, fire department and poison centre which are listed in the front of telephone books. Fill in the chart on the back cover of this manual with these numbers. Keep this manual near your telephone.

- If at all possible, never leave a casualty alone; designate someone to go for help, have them return to the scene and report to you.

WHEN CALLING FOR HELP
provide the following information:

- Your identity and a description of the accident circumstances.
- The location of the emergency. **BE EXACT**
- The number of casualties/type of injuries/condition of the casualties.
- A phone number where you can be reached.

- Give the address if the emergency is in a building and identify where the entrance is.
- Give the closest major intersection if in city or lot and concession number or grid system if in rural areas.
- Ask the operator to repeat the information you have given.
- It is important for you to wait for the other person to hang up to make sure all the necessary information has been taken.

AFTER CALLING FOR HELP- WHILE WAITING FOR THE AMBULANCE

- Make accident scene accessible to emergency personnel (i.e. elevator free for use, doors unlocked, etc.).
- Continue to monitor the casualty and watch for any changes in conditions (see page 36).
- Make the casualty comfortable and reassure.

SEE CHART FOR EMERGENCY NUMBERS ON BACK COVER OF THIS MANUAL.

Chapter 8 — Secondary Assessment

What does the First Aider do until medical aid arrives or until the casualty reaches medical aid?

FIRST AID STEPS IN A SECONDARY ASSESSMENT

After dealing with the life-threatening emergencies, carry out a complete examination of the casualty. Start at the head and move down the body to the feet. **NOT ALL INJURIES ARE OBVIOUS.**

- If casualty is conscious, **ask** what is wrong.
- **DO NOT MOVE THE CASUALTY UNNECESSARILY.** Tell the casualty what you are going to be doing and caution them not to move.
- See that no further injury occurs.
- Reassure the casualty.
- Provide covering over and under the casualty to conserve body heat and protect them from unnecessary exposure.
- Note and record any change in the casualty's condition. It is important for the First Aider to note changes which occur in the casualty. The process of noting changes requires repeated observations. **CHECK THE FOLLOWING AND RECORD ANY CHANGES:**

1. Level of Consciousness:

- Is the casualty awake and alert, or is there an altered level of consciousness, i.e. slurred speech, responds to voice, responds to pain only, or unresponsive.

2. Respiration:

- Rate of breathing
- Depth of each breath Rhythm
- Pain during respiration
- Sound of breathing: listen for raspiness or wheezing, for instance.

3. Pulse

- Rate of pulse
- Quality of pulse

4. Pupils of Eyes:

- Are they large or small?
- Are they of equal or unequal size?
- Do they react to a change in lighting?

5. Skin Colour:

- Is the casualty's skin colour: Pale
  Bluish (cyanotic) (note that in persons with darker skin pigmentation, this can be checked by examamining the inside of the mouth)
  Flushed

6. Smell (odour):

i.e. acetone breath, alcohol

Continue by carrying out a systematic examination of the casualty from head to toe. Any further injury should be sought out. This should prevent further injury resulting from the handling or transportation of the casualty to the hospital (see Table 8.1).

TABLE 8.1
SECONDARY ASSESSMENT

Location:	Check for:
Head	-bumps -blood, fluid from ears -eyes, responsiveness of pupils -breathing - changes -facial fractures
Neck	-swelling, pain -bleeding
Chest	-pain -deformity -bleeding -breathing - changes
Abdomen	-pain -swelling -discolouration (bruising)
Back	-check hollows -swelling -pain -bleeding
Pelvic Area	-pain -bleeding -swelling
Limbs	-pain -swelling or deformity -loss of sensation -symmetry -movement -colour

MEDICAL IDENTIFICATION

Anyone suffering from drug allergies or a disease needing rapid identification in an emergency, should wear some form of medical identification. (see Figure 8.1)

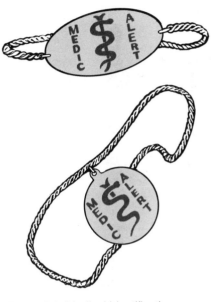

Figure 8.1: Medical Identification

Whatever the cause of an accident, check for some type of medical identification. This will be around the casualty's wrist or neck. Medical problems are identified on the back of the tag.

Also check the casualty's wallet or purse for medical information. If possible have a second person present when searching for wallet identification. Obtain that person's name, address and telephone number as well.

Chapter 9 — Head and Spinal Injuries

HEAD INJURIES

Head injuries should always be considered **SERIOUS.** They require medical attention.

TYPES OF HEAD INJURIES

LACERATION – cuts resulting from contact with a sharp object.

CONCUSSION – a shaking up or vibration of the brain from a fall or direct blow.

FRACTURE – a break in the skull caused by a blow or heavy fall.

SIGNS AND SYMPTOMS OF HEAD INJURIES

- The casualty may appear dazed, disoriented or dizzy
- Nausea or vomiting
- Drowsiness
- Possible loss of consciousness
- A noticeable change in pupil size
- Possible bleeding or clear fluid from the ear(s) and/or nose
- Headache

FIRST AID FOR HEAD INJURIES (General)

- **Always care for as a spinal injury.** Any blow to the head strong enough to cause unconsciousness may also cause a cervical spine injury.
- Immobilize the head and neck (see Figure 9.1).
- Check the casualty's breathing - look, listen and feel. If the casualty is not breathing give Rescue Breathing (see page 15-18) and CPR (see page 81) if their heart stops.
- Perform the jaw thrust to open

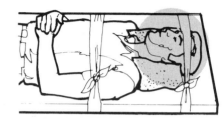

Figure 9.1: Immobilization of Head and Neck

the airway if airway is obstructed (see page 5).
- A casualty who is conscious should be advised not to move. Check with the casualty for painful areas, or loss of feeling, or movement in any part of the body. If feeling (i.e. tingling) is present, this does not mean there is no spinal injury. It simply means the spinal cord is still intact.
- If the person is bleeding from openings, like the nose, mouth or ears, do not stop the bleeding. Position the casualty to permit free drainage. Cover the wound lightly to prevent infection (see Figure 9.2).
- If bleeding occurs from facial or scalp wounds, treat it as a normal injury.
- DO NOT MOVE the casualty unless there is a danger of further injury.
- A casualty with a head injury should be under a doctor's supervision.
- Seek medical attention for the injury.
- Care for shock (see page 24).

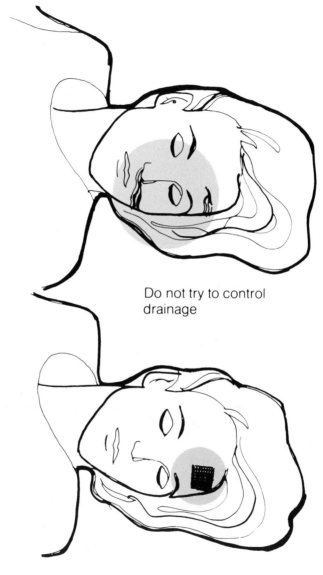

Do not try to control
drainage

Cover open wounds lightly
to prevent infection

Figure 9.2: Care for Head Injuries

SPINAL INJURIES

Over 200 bones comprise the skeleton or framework of the body. They give the body shape and they support and protect important organs. Bones are held together by ligaments. Muscles are attached to our bones with tendons. Injuries that may occur to bones or joints are called fractures, sprains, strains or dislocations.

THE SPINE

The spine is made up of a number of bones (vertebrae) joined together to form the spinal column (see Figure 9.3). Between the vertebrae are strong discs which cushion the shock of movements like walking, running, bending or jumping. The vertebrae are held together with strong muscles and ligaments and provide the delicate spinal cord with protection and support.

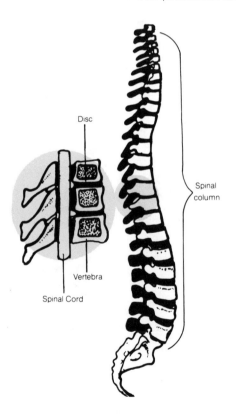

Figure 9.3: The Spinal Column and the Spinal Cord

The spinal column forms a tunnel through which the spinal cord passes. The spinal cord is nerve tissue, which is easily damaged, and if cut or torn, will never heal completely (see Figure 9.4). The cord carries messages (nerve impulses) between the brain and the body. A fracture or dislocation of one or more of the vertebrae can damage the spinal cord. Careless or rough handling of a casualty with a spinal injury, may cause serious damage to the spinal cord. **Never move anyone with a suspected spinal injury UNLESS ABSOLUTELY NECESSARY.**

CAUSES OF SPINAL INJURIES

- falls
- severe blows
- diving accidents
- motor vehicle accidents

PREVENTION IS THE FIRST STEP IN FIRST AID FOR SPINAL INJURIES

- keep stairways well lighted and uncluttered
- in winter keep outdoor steps clear of ice and snow
- NEVER DIVE into unknown waters **LOOK BEFORE YOU LEAP**
- **wear your seatbelts**

SIGNS AND SYMPTOMS OF SPINAL INJURIES

- A loss of motion and feeling below the level of injury.
- Severe pain at the point of the spinal injury.
- a tingling, "pins and needles" feeling below the level of injury.
- may be some deformation along the spinal column.

FIRST AID FOR SPINAL INJURIES

If there is even the slightest reason to suspect a neck, head or back injury, care for the casualty as a spinal injury. The following steps must be done in order:

- Reassure the casualty
- Keep casualty still
- Immobilize head, neck and back (see Figure 9.1)
- Care for shock (see page 24)
- Do a body check for other injuries, trying not to move other body parts
- Cover the casualty to maintain body temperature
- Notice and record changes (see page 36)
- Do not move the casualty unless there is further danger to the casualty or yourself
- If the casualty must be moved, ensure that they are securely held and kept still during transit (see Figure 9.5)
- Send for medical help and arrange for transportation

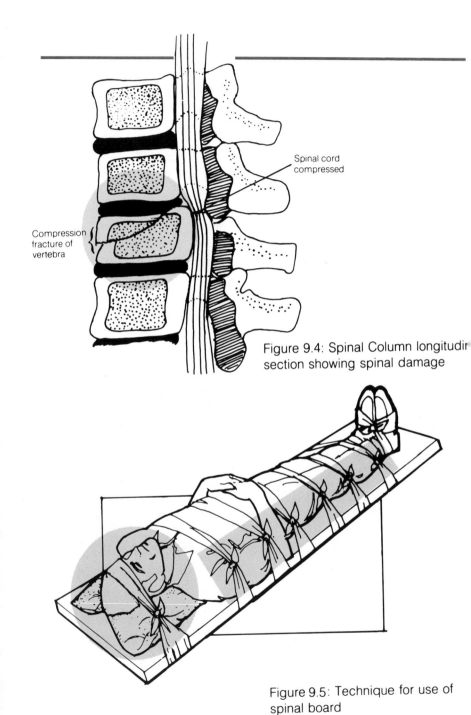

Spinal cord
compressed

Compression
fracture of
vertebra

Figure 9.4: Spinal Column longitudir
section showing spinal damage

Figure 9.5: Technique for use of
spinal board

Chapter 10 — Bone and Joint Injuries

A fracture is a break in the bone. The break may be complete or incomplete.

PREVENTION IS THE FIRST STEP IN FIRST AID FOR FRACTURES

- Always use automobile seatbelts
- Use proper equipment and be sure to warm up prior to participation in contact sports
- Assess your home for conditions which could lead to **falls**
- Train children to put toys away
- Stairways should be well lighted, clear of clutter and have sturdy handrail
- Never position small area rugs at the top or bottom of a stairway
- Always use a non-skid bathmat in the tub/shower
- Wipe up spills **immediately**
- Anchor any rug without a non-slip backing

Figure 10.1: Major types of fractures

Simple   Compound

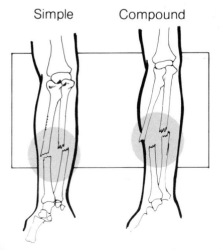

Fractures can be classified as:

1. Simple or Closed
2. Compound or Open (see Figure 10.1)

SIGNS AND SYMPTOMS OF A FRACTURE

- Painful or tender to touch
- An inability to move the injured part
- Deformity of injured body part
- Swelling and discolouration
- A shortening of a limb may be present
- Injured side of body may appear different than uninjured side.
- Casualty may report hearing a crack

Simple or Closed Fractures involve injury to the bone without disruption of the overlying skin.

Compound or Open fractures include fractures with a break in the skin over the fracture site.

Possible Causes of Fractures

- **direct force** i.e. casualty struck by an automobile may suffer a fractured leg at the point where the leg was hit by the vehicle's bumper.
- **indirect force** i.e. falls whereby a casualty lands on their hands or feet which may result in an arm or leg fracture.
- **twisting force** i.e. common to sporting accidents, a casualty's foot may be caught sufficiently to fracture one or both of the leg bones.

FIRST AID FOR FRACTURES
(General)

- Handle casualty gently.
- Stabilize the joints both above and below the fracture site. Use a splint or the casualty's body or limbs for support.
- **Always splint the fracture in the position found.**
- Support the splinted area of the upper body with a sling, if necessary
- Handle the injury carefully to avoid moving the bone and causing further damage.
- Instruct the casualty to keep the injured part still.
- If there is a compound fracture, care for the wound **before** immobilizing the fracture. (see page 55)
- Seek medical attention for the injury.
- Care for shock (see page 24).

Fractured Jaw - casualty will usually support his own jaw if able, but if he is unable to support it himself the First Aider should place the casualty in the semi-prone position and support the forehead on a rolled blanket to allow for drainage and maintenance of the airway .

Fractured Ribs-Avoid splinting. Place casualty in the most comfortable position. Stress immobility, or extreme care in moving, to avoid further tissue damage. If casualty is to be put in semi-prone position place the injured side up (for comfort) unless bleeding is occurring.

Fractured Pelvis-care for as a spinal injury. Move only with extreme care after immobilizing legs and knees. Use splint, if available, from armpits to feet. Transport on backboard. (see Figure 9.5 page 42).

SLINGS

Slings are supports for injured areas.

They help to:

- prevent further injury.
- ease pain.
- provide support.

Improvised Slings

Slings may be made on the spot using a jacket or shirt, a tie, or an uninjured body part.

The Triangular Bandage (see Figure 10.2)

The triangular bandage is usually made from factory cotton, 40 inches square, and cut diagonally to form a triangle (see figure 10.2 page 45). The bandage can be improvised from a sheet, pillow slip, shirt or any fabric which is large enough.

Types of Bandages

An Open Bandage is the full-sized triangular bandage.

A Broad Bandage is formed by taking the point to the base and then folding it again to the base.

A Narrow or Cravat Bandage is formed by folding the broad bandage once again.

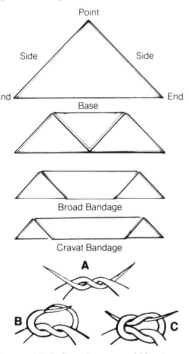

Figure 10.2: Bandages and Knots

Tying the Bandage

The ends of a bandage are fastened by a knot. A reef or square knot is preferred because it lies flat and will not slip, yet may be undone with little pain to the casualty. To tie a reef knot, place the right end over the left and around it (Figure 10.2, A). Then place the original right end-now the left end-over and around the other end (Figure 10.2

B and C). When the ends are pulled the knot is complete.

FIRST AID FOR COLLAR-BONE FRACTURE
(see Figures 10.3-10.5)

The forearm of the injured side is placed across the chest, the fingers pointing towards the opposite shoulder.

1. Place an open triangular bandage (see Figure 10.2) over the forearm and hand. The point of the bandage should extend past the elbow and shoulder.
2. Support the forearm and **ease** the bandage under the hand, forearm and elbow. Carry the lower end around the back.
3. Adjust the height of the sling, **gently.** Tie the ends together in the hollow of the neck on the **uninjured** side. Tuck the point in between the forearm and the bandage.
4. Pad between the arm and the body, in the natural hollows with soft, firm material.
5. Tie a broad bandage from the injured elbow across the body making sure the bandage is firmly in position. (Note: the pull of the broad bandage should be directed to the rear in order to keep the fractured bone ends separated.)
6. Seek medical attention for the injury.
7. Care for shock (see page 24).

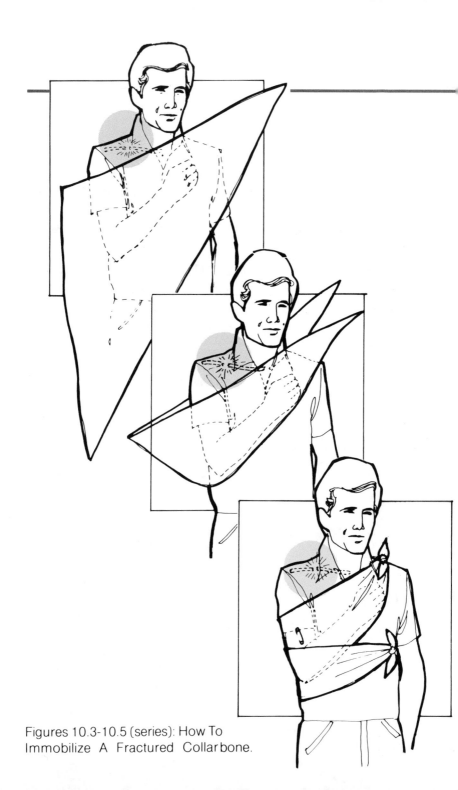

Figures 10.3-10.5 (series): How To
Immobilize A Fractured Collarbone.

UPPER ARM FRACTURES

This type of fracture occurs most frequently after a fall or a motor vehicle accident. Dislocations of the shoulder joint and sprains are also common with upper arm fractures.

FIRST AID FOR UPPER ARM FRACTURE
Use of The Small Arm Sling

The broad bandage is placed over the wrist of the injured arm with an edge at the base of the little finger. The top end is carried over the shoulder of the injured side, and around the neck onto the shoulder of the uninjured side. The other end is carried up under the wrist of the injured arm and the two ends are tied in a reef knot, which should rest in the hollow just above the collar bone on the uninjured side. The Small Arm Sling is used for injuries involving the upper arm. A broad bandage completes the immobilization (see Figures 10.6, 10.7)

- Place padding between the arm and body, in the natural hollows.
- Seek medical attention
- Care for shock (see page 24)

Figures 10.6-10.7
How To Immobilize
An Upper Arm Fracture

LOWER ARM FRACTURES

The forearm has two bones. Either bone or both bones may be broken.

FIRST AID FOR LOWER ARM FRACTURE

1. Carefully place a padded splint at the fracture site in order to stabilize the joints above and below the fracture.ᵏ This promotes comfort and provides support to the injured arm. Folded newspapers, magazines or the chestwall are excellent substitutes for a splint. (see Figures 10.8-10.10)
2. Apply a large arm sling.
3. Seek medical attention for the injury.
4. Care for shock (see page 24).

APPLICATION OF A LARGE ARM SLING
(see Figure 10.10)

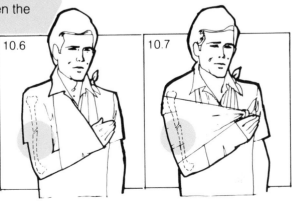

10.6   10.7

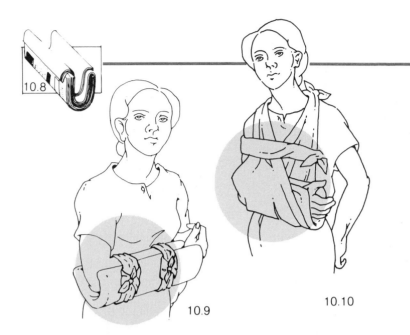

Figures 10.8-10.10: How to immobilize a lower arm fracture

The Large Arm Sling

One end of the base of a triangular bandage is placed around the neck with the end resting upon the shoulder of th uninjured side and the other end hanging loosely down in front of the casualty. The point is passed under and beyond the elbow of the injured arm. The base of the bandage should be under the tips of the fingers. The lower end is brought up and tied to the upper end with a reef knot. This knot should rest in the hollow just above the collar bone on the uninjured side. While making and tying the sling the elbow on the injured side should be kept at a right angle and the injured arm should be supported by either the casualty or a third party. The large arm sling is used for injuries involving the elbow and lower arm.

SPLINTS

A splint is an external support for an injured area of the body where a fracture is suspected. A splint steadies the injured part, thus reducing the movement of a broken bone and the joints above and below the break. It also helps prevent further tissue damage.

There are many kinds of splints, some are bought and others can be made from any object at hand, like newspapers or magazines, or even a broomstick. At times, part of the casualty's body may work as a splint.

Splints should be:

-long enough, wide enough and firm enough to hold the joints still and secure above and below the fracture.

-well padded with any available material to fit closely the shape of the body.

-secured at the top and bottom of splint and wherever else is necessary to provide support and prevent movement. (see Figure 10.11)

Application of Splints

1. Either slide the splint under the fractured area, or place it alongside the area. Make sure the splint is long enough to extend past the joints on either side of the injured area.
2. The splint should be securely fastened in place with ties, strips of cloth or bandages above and

below the injury.

3. Make the splint fit closely to the injured part by using pads.

Splints are intended to prevent the movements of an injured part of the body during transportation, whether the injury is a fractured bone, a damaged joint or severely injured soft tissues. Thin, light wooden strips can be used if they are available. If prepared splints are not at hand, they must be made by the first aider. The materials should be carefully chosen; for example pillows, a folded blanket, small boxes, corrugated cardboard or folded newspapers. If no splints are available, the First Aider's hands may be used in such a way as to hold the fracture. Every home, automobile, school and business plant should have a proper set of splints readily available.

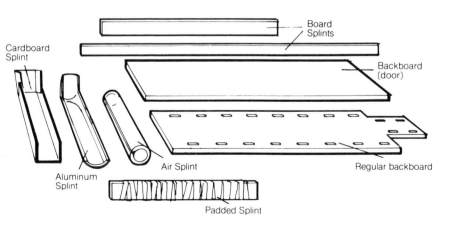

Figure 10.11: Types of Splints

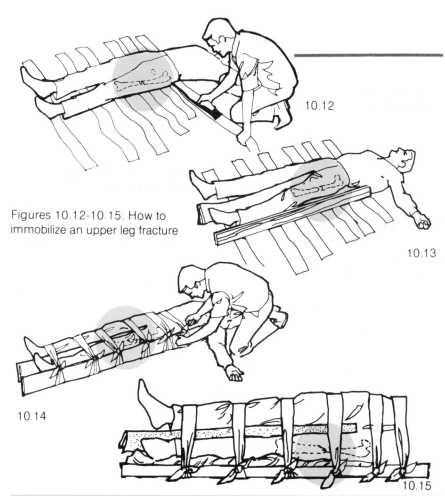

Figures 10.12-10.15: How to immobilize an upper leg fracture

10.12

10.13

10.14

10.15

FIRST AID FOR UPPER LEG FRACTURE

1. Splint the leg **in the position found.** (see Figure 10.12-10.15)
2. If there is an open wound, cover it with a sterile or clean bulky pad. Secure the dressing in place and then the splint.
3. Slide the bandages into place.
4. Padded board splints should extend from the casualty's lower chest to below the knee on the outside. Use the casualty's other leg as the splint for the inside of the leg. Place blankets or towels as packing between the legs.
5. Place the padded splint into position.
6. Place additional padding at the knees and ankles.
7. Continue by making snug ties on the outer splint.
8. Seek medical attention for the injury.
9. Care for shock (see page 24).

FIRST AID FOR LOWER LEG FRACTURE

1. Apply a well padded splint to the outside of the injured leg and foot. (see Figures 10.16-10.18) Use the uninjured leg as the other splint.
2. Place blankets or towels or any type of packing between the legs and tie the legs together securely.
3. Make sure that the splint goes above the knee.
4. Check the bandages to make sure they are not stopping circulation to the lower leg or foot.
5. Seek medical attention for the injury.
6. Care for shock (see page 24).

ANKLE OR FOOT FRACTURE

An ankle or foot fracture usually results from a fall, vehicle or sporting accident.

FIRST AID FOR ANKLE OR FOOT FRACTURE

1. Keep the casualty lying down. (see Figures 10.19-10.21).
2. If there is an open wound apply a pressure dressing to the wound.
3. Splint firmly with a pillow or as shown in Figures 10.19-10.21. **Do not try to correct any unnatural positioning. Do not remove shoe(s).**
4. Seek medical attention for the injury.

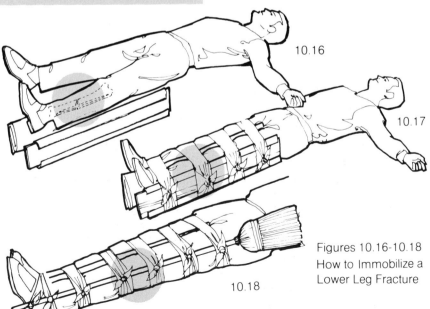

10.16

10.17

10.18

Figures 10.16-10.18
How to Immobilize a
Lower Leg Fracture

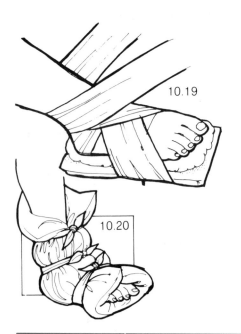

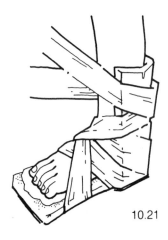

10.21
Immobilizing a fractured ankle

Figures 10.19-10.21
How to Immobilize a Fractured Foot

SPRAINS

A sprain is an injury to a joint caused by over stretching or wrenching the ligaments. A ligament is a broad band of tough fibrous tissue which connects bones together at a joint.

Most commonly affected areas are ankles and knees.

Prevention is the First Step in First Aid for Sprains, Strains and Dislocations.

When lifting:

a) always bend your knees; never stoop.

b) always stand close to an object to be lifted.

c) keep the back straight and **LIFT WITH THE LEGS.**

d) when turning never twist; take small steps and follow your feet.

In sporting activities:

a) always warm up thoroughly;

b) always wear the appropriate, correct fitting equipment.

Signs and Symptoms of a Sprain

- swelling
- pain
- discolouration (purple) bruising
- injured area may become non-functional

FIRST AID FOR SPRAINS

- Do not remove footwear; it serves as a natural splint and controls swelling.
- Apply cold pack if available to control swelling.
- Place the casualty in the most comfortable position. **Care for the injury as a fracture.**
- Seek medical attention.

STRAINS

A strain is caused by an overstretching or tearing of muscles or tendons. A common area for strains is the back, due to improper lifting.

Signs and Symptoms of a Strain

- intense pain
- swelling
- cramping may occur near the injury

Since bones and joints are not injured, they should remain functional in strains.

FIRST AID FOR STRAINS

- Place the casualty in a comfortable position.
- Immobilize and care for the injury as a fracture.
- Apply a cold compress.
- Seek medical attention for the injury.

DISLOCATIONS

A dislocation occurs when a bone becomes out of place at a joint. It is usually caused by a fall or blow, forcing a joint into an unnatural position.

Signs and Symptoms of Dislocations

- signs and symptoms are generally the same as for fractures
- unnatural position and appearance of the injured joint
- pain
- swelling
- loss of normal movement at the joint

FIRST AID FOR DISLOCATIONS

- Care for the injury in the position it is found.
- Securely splint and support with a sling.
- Care for the injury as a fracture.
- Do not attempt to return the bone to its proper position.
- Seek medical attention for the injury.

Chapter 11 — Wounds

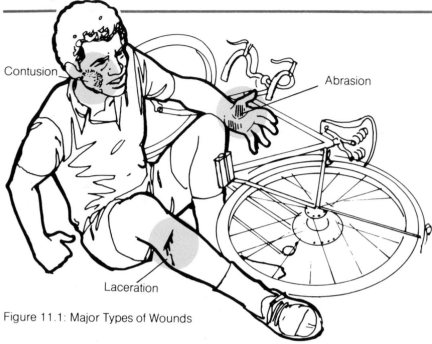

Figure 11.1: Major Types of Wounds

A wound is an injury to soft tissues, such as the skin or mucous membranes. The possibility of infection exists with all wounds.

TYPES OF WOUNDS

CONTUSION-bruising, without a break in the skin.

ABRASIONS-surface injuries like scratches and scrapes.

PUNCTURE WOUNDS-small diameter, often deep injuries from pointed objects.

CRUSHING WOUNDS-deep injuries causing structural damage, like bone fractures.

LACERATION-cut or tear caused by objects like broken bottles (see Figure 11.1).

PREVENTION OF WOUNDS

Prevention is the First Step in First Aid for Wounds.

- use protective clothing or equipment if participating in any high risk situation (e.g. sports, workshop, garden).
- store sharp objects such as knives out of reach of children.
- when using knives, always carve away from your body and fingers.

Signs and Symptoms of Wounds

- bleeding
- pain
- discolouration of the area

FIRST AID FOR WOUNDS

- If possible, first aiders should wash their hands.
- If running water is available, gently cleanse the injured area, wiping away from the wound, to remove surface dirt. For large wounds wash away the dirt, and bring the edges of the wound together and securely apply a dressing or bandage to cover the area.

- The danger of tetanus (lockjaw) should be considered with all wounds, not only with deeply penetrating or puncture wounds.
- Suggest that the casualty seek medical attention for immunization.
- Care for shock (see page 24).
- Bruises or contusions in which the underlying tissue is damaged and the outer skin is unbroken should be cared for immediately. Apply cold to the bruised area in the form of an ice pack, cold water or snow to decrease swelling or pain.

NOTE: Do not put snow, or cold compresses directly on a wound. Place a layer of clean material between the cold item and bruised area. Never judge the seriousness of a wound by the size of the puncture hole.

Wounds that involve deep penetration into the body, such as abdominal wounds, require immediate professional medical care. In such cases the First Aider should attempt to prevent infection and control bleeding by covering the area with a dressing and reassuring the casualty while professional transportation and/or medical aid is sought. A casualty with a chest injury should be placed in a semi-prone position with the injured side down to facilitate drainage and easier breathing.

ANIMAL BITES

Animal bites are usually lacerations or puncture wounds and a First Aider should care for them like any other wound of this type. However, there is always a danger of tetanus and/or rabies, so the casualty should have medical attention. The general location of the attacking animal should be noted and reported to police because of rabies threat. The animal should be quaranteened until the local health authorities are notified, or if it is certain the animal has had an up-to-date rabies vacination.

BLOOD SUCKERS/LEECHES

Blood suckers or leeches may attach themselves to your skin while you are wading or swimming.

FIRST AID FOR BLOOD SUCKERS/LEECHES

- To remove suckers or leeches, first sprinkle them with salt and then rub them with dry sand.
- Wash the wound area with soap and water.

TICKS

Ticks attach themselves to the base of hairs or to the skin with their mouthparts.

FIRST AID FOR TICKS

- Cover the area with mineral oil or vaseline to cut off the air supply and within half an hour the tick will usually let go. Application of acetone or nail polish remover is also effective.
- It is important to ensure that all parts of the tick are removed. Forcible removal may leave some part under the skin, possibly causing infection. Use tweezers to remove any remaining parts.

- Wash with soap and water.
- If a fever or rash ensues in the casualty within the next 10 days seek medical attention immediately. Tick fever can be fatal.

INSECT BITES

Insect bites may cause discomfort but are usually harmless.

SIGNS AND SYMPTOMS OF INSECT BITES

- A swelling in the bite area.
- Pain and itchiness.

FIRST AID FOR INSECT BITES

- Look for medical identification (bracelet, necklace, wallet card).
- Apply a cold compress, then apply a soothing lotion such as calamine to the injured area.
- If an acute swelling occurs, seek medical attention.

SNAKE BITE

PREVENTION IS THE FIRST STEP IN FIRST AID FOR SNAKE BITE.

Snakes usually prefer shaded areas, such as rockpits, swamps, undergrowth, or abandoned shacks and hay lofts. When in these areas, wear leather boots, stockings, long sleeves and gloves. When rock climbing, do not place your fingers into ledges you haven't inspected. Carry a snake bite kit.

Facts about snakes:

- Most snakes in Canada are non-poisonous. They will bite if provoked. The bite should be treated as a simple wound.
- The most common group of venomous snakes in Canada are rattlesnakes. Other groups are the copperhead and water moccasin. When in areas with poisonous snakes, carry a snake bite kit.
- You may not hear the rattle of a snake's tail before it strikes.
- Snakes strike mainly at moving objects.
- The striking range of a snake is about two-thirds of its length forward and one-third upward. If you are out of range, and see the snake, carefully step backwards to a safe area.
- Snakes swim well and their bite underwater is as effective as on land. In water, snakes have a shorter striking range.
- Snakes do not hear, but they do detect vibrations. Therefore, if you are within striking range **do not yell.**

SIGNS AND SYMPTOMS OF SNAKE BITES

- Pain (if bite poisonous, pain may be extreme.)
- One or more puncture wounds.
- A discoloration and swelling in the bitten area.
- Weakness, difficulty in breathing, gradual loss of consciousness and possible death if the bite is not cared for.

FIRST AID FOR SNAKE BITES

- Place the casualty at rest and **lower** the bitten area below the level of the heart, if practical, to slow the absorption of venom.
- Reassure the casualty, and advise the person not to walk or move around.
- Death from a snake bite rarely occurs but the casualty should receive medical assistance as soon as possible. Due to their small body mass, the risk is greater with small children.
- Make sure a casualty who is having difficulty in breathing has an open airway and if the casualty stops breathing begin Rescue Breathing (see page 14-18) and CPR (see page 81) if their heart stops.
- Seek immediate medical attention for the casualty.

BANDAGING TECHNIQUES FOR WOUNDS

Bandaging for Head Wounds

Fold a narrow hem along the base of an open bandage. Place the centre of the base immediately above the eyebrows, with the point passed over the head to the back of the neck. Carry the ends around the head, passing them above the ears and crossing behind the head well under the base of the skull. Carry the ends to the front of the head and tie on the forehead over the base of the bandage. The point of the bandage should be pulled down snugly and then pinned up over the dressing.

Bandaging for Chest or Back Wounds

Place the point of the bandage over one shoulder allowing the open bandage to hang over the chest. Carry the ends around the trunk and body tying them so the knot is located below the shoulder on which the point is resting. There will be one long end left after the knot is tied. Carry this end up to the shoulder and tie it there.

Bandaging for Hand Wounds

Fold a narrow hem along the base of an open bandage. Place the injured hand on the bandage with the dressing uppermost so that the fingers are directed toward the point and the wrist is on the centre of the base. Carry the point of the bandage over the hand and place it on the forearm. Cross the ends and carry them around the wrist. Tie the ends together. Fold the point over the knot and secure it.

Bandaging for Knee Wounds

Place an open triangular bandage over the injured knee with the point on the upper part of the thigh. Fold a narrow hem along the base of the bandage and carry the ends around the leg, below the knee. Cross the ends behind the knee and carry them around to the front of the thigh (above the knee) and tie. Fold the point down over the knot and secure it.

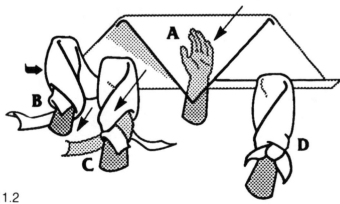

Figure 11.2
Hand Bandaging

Chapter 12 — Injuries Due to Heat or Cold

Burns

Burns are tissue injuries resulting from over-exposure to excessive heat. Possible sources of heat include: thermal (like fire or steam), chemical (like lye or acids), electrical (electricity) or radiation (sun) sources.

PREVENTION IS THE FIRST STEP IN FIRST AID FOR BURNS.

• Never let pot handles protrude while on the stove.
• Lift the far edge of lids on hot pans first to prevent burns from steam.
• Ensure flammables and matches are appropriately stored away from children.
• Special care should always be taken while smoking.
• Don't leave children alone during food preparation.
• All electrical cords should be kept clear of counter edges since toddlers use these as ropes, causing appliances to be pulled down on them.
• Double check before leaving the kitchen to ensure burners are turned off.
• Keep curtains, clothing etc. at a safe distance from fireplaces and stoves.

Rescue Procedures

If escaping from a burning building:

a. Feel doors for heat.
b. Keep doors closed; if hot, **do not open.** Find some other means of reaching safety.
c. Cover your nose and mouth with damp cloths to cool inhaled air. Stay near windows where the air will be cooler and purer, but keep windows closed.
d. Move near the floor on hands and knees where the air is cooler and purer.
e. If you become trapped, and the only exit is a window, do not panic and jump. Wait for rescue or attempt to exit by sliding down knotted sheets or a rope. If you must drop from a window shorten the distance by hanging full length from the sill before releasing your grip.
f. Encourage trapped persons not to jump. Organized rescue operations take time. Throw a rope to the window or put up a ladder. Instruct the person to tie the sheets or rope to an object that will not pull out of the window, such as a bed or radiators.

Types of Burns (see Figure 12.1)

• **1ST degree burn**-redness. This is a minor burn, but can be very painful.

• **2ND degree burn**-redness and formation of blisters. This is a severe burn and can be life-threatening if a large area of the body is involved. The burn is painful but should heal with little scarring. They are usually caused by scalding or a brief flash of heat.

59

- **3RD degree burn**-charred, blackened appearance. This can be a life-threatening injury. It poses a definite threat of infection. There will be less pain at first because of severe nerve damage.

These burns are usually caused by flame.

Medical and surgical help is necessary, healing is slow, and dense scars will form.

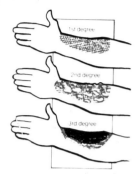

Figure 12.1
Major Types of Burns

the chemical is removed, diluted or neutralized immediately.

FIRST AID FOR BURNS

1st Degree
- Immerse the burned area in cool water at once.

2nd Degree
- Immerse the burned area in cool water at once, unless the burn is extensive, i.e. involves body and extremities.
- Do not break blisters; **these are "nature's bandages".**
- If the blisters break, care for the injury as a wound.
- Seek medical attention.
- Treat for shock (see page 24).

3rd Degree
- Apply cool **clean** water to cool the burned area.
- Cover the entire burn lightly with a lint-free cloth.
- Seek medical attention immediately for the injury.
- Treat for shock (see page 24).

CHEMICAL BURNS

Chemical burns to the skin or to the eyes require special care to ensure

FIRST AID FOR CHEMICAL BURNS

- If the chemical is in powder form, brush away with a clean cloth before flushing.
- Ensure that no other person including yourself will be contaminated with the removed chemical.
- Use a forceful spray of cool, clean water for a long period to dilute the chemical. Water should be avoided in chemical burns from any metals, such as sodium, potassium, magnesium, and aluminum. Mineral oil may be used to cover chemical metal burns.

Do not waste time looking for an antidote.

- Remove any contaminated clothing from the casualty.
- Seek medical attention for the burn.

EYE BURNS

Eye burns can result from extreme heat, chemical splash, over-exposure to sun, snow glare, or a solar eclipse.

FIRST AID FOR EYE BURNS
For chemical splash burn:
- Flush the eye(s) with large amounts of water for at least 10 minutes including under eye lids from the inside to the outside. Ensure the drainage from the burned eye does not run into the other eye.
- Have casualty blink constantly while flushing, to get under lid. DO NOT LIFT THE LIDS.
- Loosely bandage both eyes to cut down on eye movement.
- Seek medical attention for the burn.

For over-exposure to heat or glare:
- Loosely bandage both eyes.
- Use cool wet packs to relieve pain.
- Seek medical attention.

FIRST AID FOR ELECTRICAL BURNS
- Electrical contact with the skin and body can result in serious injury.
- Electrical burns have an entrance and exit wound, with internal damage in between.
- Carefully remove the source of contact or the casualty from the source - **Do not directly touch the casualty if the source is still present.**
- Check airway, breathing and circulation.
- Treat as a third-degree burn (see page 60).
- Care for shock (see page 24).

SUNBURN (Radiation)

Sunburn is caused by over-exposure to ultraviolet radiation, either from the sun or sunlamps. It can produce first or second degree burns.

Signs and Symptoms of Sunburn
- Colouring may vary from slight to intense redness.
- Blistering of the skin may follow.
- Pain and inability to move the burned areas can develop.
- There may be symptoms of heat stroke or heat exhaustion.

FIRST AID FOR SUNBURN
- Move out of sunlight.
- Care for the burn injury according to degree of damage.
- Apply soothing lotion to the burn.
- If heat exhaustion or heat stroke symptoms appear, treat as shown (see page 61 and 62).

HEAT EXHAUSTION

Heat exhaustion results from exposure or extensive physical activity in high temperatures and/or high humidity, causing loss of body fluids and chemicals.

Signs of Heat Exhaustion
- Weakness, dizziness
- Nausea and vomiting
- Pale, clammy skin
- Rapid breathing
- Perspiration may appear on forehead and face

FIRST AID FOR HEAT EXHAUSTION

- Move the casualty to a cool, shady area.
- Care for shock.
- If the casualty complains of chilliness, cover lightly.
- Replace lost fluids by giving sips of cool water.
- Cool the person gradually by putting in a cool area, remove as much clothing as possible, sponge the body with tepid water, and fan either by hand or mechanically.

HEAT STROKE

Heat stroke results from overexposure to sunlight and an individual's inability to lower their body temperature. This can be a life-threatening situation if it is not cared for immediately.

Signs and Symptoms of Heat Stroke

- Restlessness, bizarre behaviour.
- Headache, nausea and vomiting
- Hot, flushed skin which is red and often dry.
- High body temperature.
- If not cared for the casualty will lose consciousness

FIRST AID FOR HEAT STROKE

- Check the casualty's breathing, and pulse.

- Move the person to a cool, shady area.
- Place cold compresses around the casulaty's head, along the sides of the chest and in the armpits.
- Place ice packs to the armpits and groin.
- Remove clothes, sponge with tepid water, and fan either by hand or mechanically.
- If the casualty is conscious and not nauseated you may provide sips of cool fluids.
- Seek medical attention.

PREVENTION IS THE FIRST STEP IN FIRST AID FOR INJURIES DUE TO COLD

1. Avoid tight gloves, socks and footwear.
2. Change damp socks or gloves.
3. Maintain circulation by moving your toes, stamping your feet and swinging your arms.
4. Stay dry. Put on rain gear before you get wet. The body loses heat 200 times faster if your clothes are wet.
5. Cover your head and neck to reduce heat loss. Up to 60% of body heat loss can occur through an uncovered head.
6. Wool is warmer than cotton or synthetics and retains much of

its warmth even when wet.
7. Never ignore shivering.
8. Stay out of the wind.
9. **Do not consume alcohol;** it will increase surface circulation and cause a lower body temperature.

HYPOTHERMIA

Hypothermia is the lowering of deep body (core) temperature that depresses normal body functions.

Progressive Signs and Symptoms of Hypothermia

1. Lack of fine body coordination, e.g. use of hands.
2. Stumbling.
3. The casualty feels chilled and weary.
4. Vision becomes blurred and hallucinations may occur.
5. Uncontrollable shivering.
6. Vague, slow, slurred speech.
7. Lapses in memory.
8. The casualty may be overcome by a strong desire to sleep. This can be followed with unconsciousness and may lead to death if not cared for immediately.

FIRST AID FOR HYPOTHERMIA

The type of rewarming necessary depends on the degree of hypothermia evident. Often it is difficult to measure inner body temperature; therefore the following guidelines estimate the degree of hypothermia based on the signs and symptoms evident in the casualty.

MILD HYPOTHERMIA

If the casualty is conscious, talking clearly and sensibly and shivering vigorously then the following steps should be taken:

- All hypothermic casualties should be handled gently, avoiding jolts that might adversely affect the heart's function.
- Get them to a dry, sheltered area.
- DO NOT RUB THE SURFACE OF THE BODY.
- Remove wet clothing. If possible put on layers of dry clothing. Cover the head and neck (hat/scarf).
- Apply warm (40-45°C) objects such as water bottles, chemical heat packs, (hand warmers) when possible, to head, neck, and trunk. BE CAREFUL TO AVOID BURNS.

- Give warm drinks for mild hypothermic cases; **NEVER ALCOHOL.**

SEVERE HYPOTHERMIA

If the casualty is getting stiff and is either unconscious or showing signs of clouded consciousness such as slurred speech, or any other apparent signs of deterioration, shivering may be reduced or absent; immediately transport to medical assistance where aggressive rewarming can be initiated. **Once shivering has stopped, it is no use wrapping the casualty in blankets if there is no source of heat. This merely keeps them cold.** A way must be found to donate heat to the casualty as quickly as possible.

The following are some methods that have been used in different situations to deliver heat to the severely hypothermic casualty.

- Donate heat to the trunk of the body by direct body contact, especially to the chest, with warm person(s). The rescuer should remove their upper clothing and huddle with the casualty inside blankets/ sleeping bags.
- Apply warm (40-45°C) objects same as for mild hypothermia.
- Rescue Breathing if casualty's breathing has stopped, and CPR (see page 81) if their heart has stopped.

FROST-NIP

Frost-nip is a superficial injury caused by freezing a small area such as the nose, cheek, fingers or toes.

Signs and Symptoms of Frost-Nip

- Possible pain or stinging in the frost-nipped area followed by numbness.
- Area may appear whiter than the surrounding tissue.

FIRST AID FOR FROST NIP

- Warm the area by steady firm pressure with a warm hand.
- Blow hot breath on the area.
- Hold frost-nipped area such as fingers against the body (i.e. in armpits).
- After thawing the area, there will be a burning sensation, redness, pain and tenderness. Blisters may form, but they should not be opened.
- NO NOT RUB the frost-nipped area.

FROST-BITE

Frost-bite is the freezing of deeper body tissues by a longer period of exposure to cold. Frost-bite may be associated with hypothermia. Frost-bite always damages tissue.

Signs and Symptoms of Frost-Bite

- A waxy, white appearance in the frost-bitten area.
- In superficial frost-bite, the skin and tissues are still pliable.
- In deep frost-bite, the flesh is hard and solid to the touch.
- Joints stiffen.
- Loss of sensation.

FIRST AID FOR FROST-BITE

- Assist the casualty to the nearest shelter.
- Do not rub frozen parts.
- **Do not apply snow.**
- If there is any chance that a frozen part may be re-frozen, "DO NOT THAW IT".
- Thawing is a very painful and often requires narcotic pain medication. It is recommended the thawing be done under medical supervision, unless this will be delayed.
- To protect blisters loosely apply a dry dressing. Do not break the blisters.

NOTE:

If you must thaw a frozen part, use a container of warm water (42°C) (a comfortable temperature when tested with your elbow). The container should be large enough to immerse the frozen part. Warm the frozen area until it is completely flushed red with blood. Ensure the part does not become frozen again.

Chapter 13 — Injuries to Specific Body Areas

THE EYE

Objects such as dirt, sand, glass, and metal may become lodged in the surface of the eyeball.

Signs and Symptoms of Eye Injury

- A scratchy sensation which increases with eye movement.
- Tears forming uncontrollably.
- A sensitivity to light.

FIRST AID FOR THE EYE

- Instruct the casualty not to rub the injured eye.
- Do not attempt to remove a foreign body which has penetrated the surface of the eyeball.
- Cover both the casualty's eyes, to reduce eye movement.
- If a foreign body has penetrated the eyeball, no pressure should be applied to the eye or eyelids. Try to cover with a protective shield that does not touch the eye (small paper cup, etc.).
- Seek medical attention for the injury.

Note: Tears can wash a foreign body from the eye. The eye may still feel sensitive and irritated for a short time after. Cover the eye with a light weight bandage until any discomfort has eased.

In the case of a casualty who is wearing contact lenses, the lenses should be left alone. Make a note that contact lenses are present and seek medical attention immediately.

NOSE

The most common injuries to the nose are caused by insertion of foreign objects, usually by children, or nose bleeds resulting from an injury or medical condition.

FIRST AID FOR NOSE BLEED

- Have the casualty sit in an upright position, head forward.
- Pinch the nose firmly with thumb and forefinger on either side, where the nasal bone and cartilage meet. Hold firmly for 10 minutes or more to allow clot to form.
- The casualty's nose should not be blown for at least two hours, otherwise the clot may be disturbed and the bleeding resume.
- If bleeding continues seek medical attention.

FOREIGN OBJECTS

- If an object is in the nose and is readily seen and easily grasped, it may be removed **gently.** If the object is well inside the nose, do not use an instrument or your finger to remove it.
- Seek medical attention for the injury.

EAR

Injuries such as lacerations and bruises may be cared for like any wound. Foreign bodies in the ear, such as seeds, beans and buttons are sometimes inserted by children and require specific care.

FIRST AID FOR THE EAR

- If a foreign object is readily seen and easily grasped, it may be removed **gently.**
- If the object sticks in the ear, do not use an instrument or your fingers to remove it.
- Do not attempt to flush any object(s) from the ear, as these may swell and cause cause further damage (i.e. especially seeds and beans).
- Seek medical attention for the obstruction.

Chapter 14 — Medical Conditions

HEART ATTACKS

The actual cause of a heart attack is lack of blood and oxygen to the heart muscle. Heart attacks may result from a loss of blood supply to the heart due to either a block in one of the blood vessels supplying the heart or an interruption of the electrical stimulus within the heart wall.

Signs and Symptoms of Heart Attacks

- Heavy crushing pressure, squeezing, fullness, burning or pain in the centre of the chest sometimes extending to the shoulder, arm, neck and jaw. (see Figure 14.1).
- Vomiting and nausea.
- Headaches.
- Cold, clammy skin.
- Sweating.
- Paleness or a bluish colouration of the skin (cyanosis).
- The casualty may provide excuses for illness (denial of possible heart problems is common)
- Gasping and difficulty in breathing. The casualty may stop breathing in extreme circumstances.
- Extreme general weakness and restlessness in the casualty.
- The casualty may feel apprehensive.
- The casualty may think he is suffering from indigestion.
- Unconsciousness.

THE CASUALTY MAY HAVE SOME OR ALL OF THE ABOVE SIGNS AND SYMPTOMS IN VARYING DEGREES.

NOTE: pain may subside and return. The casualty may not necessarily look ill. 60% of deaths due to heart attack occur outside the hospital within two hours after the onset of signals. Seek medical attention, immediately.

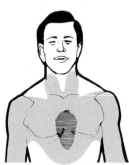 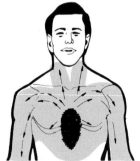 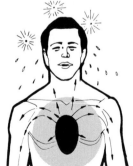

Pressure, crushing or squeezing in centre of chest.

Discomfort spreads across chest, to either shoulder and/or arm, sometimes includes neck and jaw region.

Sweating begins with nausea, vomiting difficulty breathing, faint feeling.

Figure 14.1: Early Warning Signs of Heart Attack

FIRST AID FOR HEART ATTACK

- Ensure the casualty has a clear airway.
- A casualty who is conscious should be placed in a comfortable position.
- Loosen tight clothing.
- Reassure the casualty.
- Keep the casualty quiet.
- Assist the casualty in taking medication if a prescription is at hand.
- Look for medical identification.
- If the casualty stops breathing give Rescue Breathing (see page 15-18).
- If the casualty's pulse stops CPR should be administered (see page 81).
- Seek medical attention immediately.

STROKE

A stroke (Cerebrovascular accident, CVA) occurs when the blood supply to a part of the brain is interrupted. This injures the brain cells which lie beyond the point of interruption.

Signs and Symptoms of Stroke

- Paralysis or weakness in the limbs on one side of the body.
- The casualty may have slurred speech or be unable to speak.
- The casualty may have difficulty breathing or swallowing.
- The corner of the mouth on the affected side usually droops.
- There can be loss of bladder and bowel control.
- Pupils are usually of equal size.
- The casualty may lose consciousness.
- If any of these signs and symptoms occur but later disappear — seek medical attention.

FIRST AID FOR STROKE

- Maintain an open airway.
- Place the casualty in a semi-prone position, resting on the **affected** side to aid in drainage of the mouth.
- Do not give the casualty anything which is taken through the mouth.
- Reassure the casualty.
- If the casualty stops breathing give Rescue Breathing (see page 15-18) and CPR (see page 81) if their heart has stopped.
- Seek medical attention for the casualty.

FAINTING

Fainting is a loss of consciousness due to temporary lack of blood flow to the brain.

Signs and Symptoms of Fainting

(Note: All of these signs and symptoms may be exhibited in any one casualty)

Fainting may be preceded by:

- paleness
- sweating
- dizziness
- nausea

FIRST AID FOR FAINTING

- To prevent a collapse, have the casualty lie down and elevate the feet.
- Loosen tight clothing.
- Do not attempt to raise a casualty who has collapsed. A slight elevation of the feet will speed recovery by increasing the blood supply to the head.
- Place an unconscious person in a semi-prone position (see page 25).
- If there is no recovery in 4-6 minutes, the casualty has not fainted. There may be a more serious problem.
- Maintain an open airway and seek medical help.

CONVULSION

A loss of consciousness accompanied by involuntary contraction and relaxation of major body muscles. The causes include medical conditions such as: epilepsy, drug poisoning, high fever (in infants and young children) and head injury.

Signs and Symptoms of Convulsions

During the convulsions

- The casualty may become rigid or have violent jerking movements of the body.
- There may be foaming or drooling from the mouth.

After the convulsions:

- The casualty may feel disoriented and drowsy.
- There may be a loss of consciousness for either a short or indefinite period of time, depending on the exact cause.

FIRST AID FOR CONVULSIONS

- Protect the casualty from self-injury, especially of the head.
- Do not attempt to restrain body movements more than is necessary to protect the casualty.
- Make sure the casualty's airway is open.
- Put **nothing** in the casualty's mouth.
- If the casualty's breathing stops, give Rescue Breathing after the convulsions have stopped. Be sure to check pulse and give CPR (see page 81) if necessary.
- Check for medical identification.
- Seek medical attention for the casualty.

EPILEPSY

Epilepsy is a condition manifested by seizures which are caused by an abnormal focus of activity within the brain, that produces severe motor responses or changes in consciousness. Epilepsy is a relatively common condition controlled most often by medication.

Signs and Symptoms of Epilepsy

- The casualty may cry out and then fall to the ground.
- The convulsive movements affect many muscles of the body.

FIRST AID FOR EPILEPSY

- Protect the casualty from injury on surrounding objects.
- Protect the casualty's head.
- Do not restrain the casualty during the convulsion.
- **Put nothing in the casualty's mouth.**
- When the seizure is over, place the person in semi-prone position and ensure an open airway. (see page 25)
- Watch the casualty; other seizures may occur.
- Seek medical attention.

DIABETES

A casualty in a diabetic crisis will be suffering from too much or too little sugar in the blood. Most diabetics carry medic alerts and often sugar or candy.

FIRST AID FOR DIABETIC CRISIS

- Check casualty for medical identification.
- If the casualty is conscious give sugar, candy or fruit juices.
- Make sure an unconscious casualty has an open airway.
- **Do not give insulin.**
- Seek medical attention immediately.

DIABETES

TYPES OF DIABETIC CRISIS

Signs	Insulin Shock (needs sugar)	Diabetic Coma (needs insulin)
Respirations	Shallow	Deep, sighing
State of Consciousness	Faintness to unconsciousness, may develop quickly	Gradual onset of coma
Skin	pale, sweating	Flushed, dry
Breath Odour	Odourless	Musty apple, nail polish (acetone) smell
Other Signs	Headache, Trembling, Confusion, Aggressive behaviour (sometimes)	

HIGH FEVER

An oral temperature over 39°C (102°F) should cause concern and requires medical consultation. A luke-warm sponge bath may also be given to the casualty to temporarily reduce the high fever. In young children a high fever may cause convulsions.

CHILDBIRTH

First Aiders should remember that the vast majority of deliveries are **normal, natural processes** with few complications. If delivery is imminent and there is not enough time to move the woman to a hospital; do the following:

FIRST AID FOR CHILDBIRTH

- Get a helper to call a doctor and an ambulance.
- Try to make sure at least one woman is present; this will help make the pregnant woman feel more comfortable.
- Place the woman on her back or side, whichever is most comfortable for her. If it is necessary to move her, she should walk with the help of the First Aider.
- Ensure privacy.
- Cleanliness in all aspects of childbirth is important. Wash your hands before and after the birth.

Safe Handling of the Baby

- Support the infant's head during delivery. The baby's head will turn to one side or the other. This enables the shoulders to be delivered.

Maintain support for the child.

- Support the head and neck while the trunk is delivered.
- Wipe the baby's face and mouth gently with a clean cloth to clear the nose and mouth.
- Support the baby on your forearm with feet elevated to drain the nose and throat passages (i.e. hold the baby as you would if you were about to administer Rescue Breathing (see page 17).
- Wrap the baby in clean material and dry well, then place the child on the mother's abdomen.
- Lay the baby on his/her side facing away from mother.
- Keep the mother and baby warm.
- Do not wash the baby; there is a protective coating which should not yet be removed.

Cord and After-birth:

- Handle them as little as possible.
- Do not pull at them.
- The cord and placenta will usually be expelled within 20 minutes.
- Let them drop onto a clean towel
- **DO NOT CUT THE CORD.**

- There should be no cause for alarm if the placenta is not expelled.
- Reassure the mother and interfere as little as possible.
- Ensure the baby is breathing and kept warm.
- The placenta should be saved. It should be wrapped separately but kept with the child.

Chapter 15 — Moving and Transportation

PREPARATION FOR TRANSPORT

The Cardinal Rule for Transportation:

Do not move a casualty unless it is absolutely necessary. If, however, professional transport is not available, the casualty may have to be immobilized and transported.

Moving and transportation include the safe movement of an injured person away from further danger, and the transfer to medical care. The former may have to be done by the First Aider; the latter, if at all possible, should be done by professional rescue personnel (ambulance or medical personnel) using proper equipment.

Preparation for emergency services transport:

- **Information-**Have as much information about the casualty and cause of accident as possible.

- **Changes-**All changes in the casualty's condition should be recorded and attached to casualty before transport (see page 36).

- **Causes-**If the accident is a poisoning, the poison container or a sample of the casualty's vomitus should go with the casualty.

Indications for Immediate Movement

Environmental Dangers:

- Fire, danger of fire or explosion.
- Lack of oxygen from gases or fumes (asphyxia).
- Risk of drowning.
- Possibility of collapsing walls, buildings.
- Danger of electrocution on nearby live wires.
- Traffic hazards.
- Dangers from machinery.

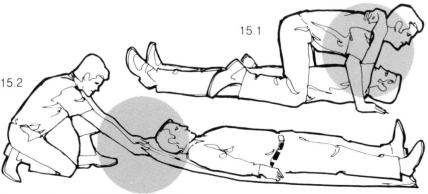

15.1

15.2

Figures 15.1 and 15.2: The Drag Carry

The Drag Carry (see Figures 15.1 and 15.2)

- If a stretcher is not available substitutes such as a blanket may be used to drag or carry a casualty. It is also possible to improvise

stretchers (see Figure 15.7).

- This method is most appropriate for short distances over smooth surfaces.

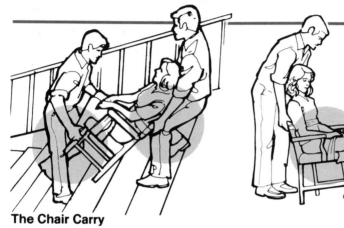

Figure 15.3: The Chair Carry

The Chair Carry

- This is effective when it is necessary to carry a casualty down narrow stairways. Make sure the chair is strong enough. (see Figure 15.3)

- Ensure that the casualty's arms and legs are secured before proceeding.

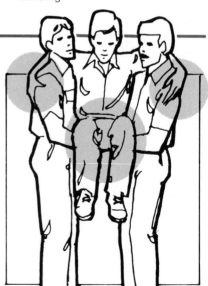

The Hand Seat This method is best used to move a conscious casualty over a short, flat distance (see Fig. 15.4-15.5).
- The procedure requires two people to transport the casualty.
- The seat may be formed by using the hook lock, the wrist lock, the two-hand seat, three hand-seat or four-hand seat.

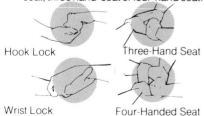

Hook Lock   Three-Hand Seat

Wrist Lock   Four-Handed Seat

Figures 15.4 and 15.5: The Hand Seat

The Human Crutch
(see Figure 15.6)

- The Human Crutch is the most useful technique for slight injuries to the lower extremities.
- Stand on the injured side of the casualty. Place your arm around the person's waist, grasping the clothing on the uninjured side.
- Pass the casualty's arm around your neck. Grasp the wrist or hand of that arm firmly with your free hand.
- Instruct the casualty to use your body as a crutch.

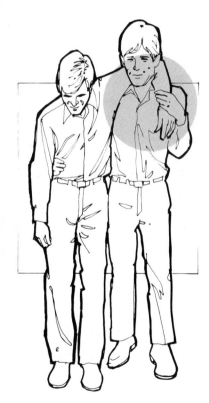

Figure 15.6: The Human Crutch

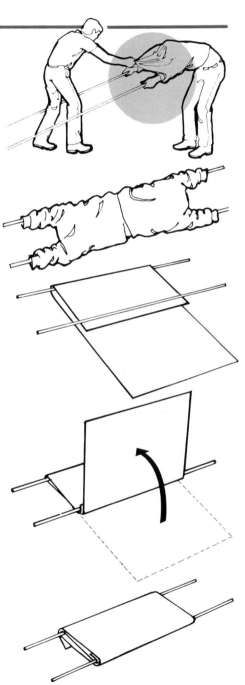

Figure 15.7: Improvised Stretchers

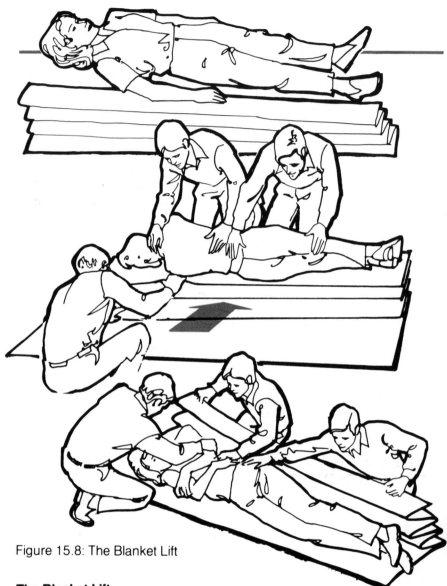

Figure 15.8: The Blanket Lift

The Blanket Lift

From the side, place a blanket under casualty. Allow about two-thirds of the blanket to fall in folds or pleats beside the casualty. Place the folded (not rolled) portion snugly against the person's body. Grasp the casualty at the hips and shoulders and gently roll their body about one-eighth of a turn away from the blanket. Push the folded part of the blanket as far under the casualty as is possible. Then roll the casualty back over the folds and about one-eighth of a turn in the opposite direction. Pull the blanket, then the sides can be rolled. The casualty can now be lifted onto a stretcher or carried to safety.

An Unconscious Casualty

- Close attention should be made to keep the casualty's airway open. Make sure fluids (mucous, vomitus) drain from the mouth by positioning the casualty in either a semi-prone position, or with the head turned to one side assuming no other injuries, e.g. spinal.
- Straps or some other restraining device should be used to prevent the casualty from falling or rolling off a stretcher.

Transportation of Spinal Injury

Casualties should only be moved if it is absolutely necessary. A special technique is required: the rescue group leader will instruct one person to apply tension to the head, another to the feet.

The leader will position people on one side of casualty, having them all kneel on the same knee.

- The leader will instruct his assistants to pass their hands over the casualty's body at the neck, chest, hips and ankles.
- At a given signal from the leader, the casualty will be rolled toward the assistants and supported there.
- A flat (non-metal) board will now be placed on the ground below the casualty.
- The leader now will give the signal to lower the casualty onto the board. When the casualty is secured, the tension is released. (see Figure 9.5 page 42).

- **TENSION MUST BE MAINTAINED AT ALL TIMES DURING MOVEMENT**

Chapter 16 — Cardiopulmonary Resuscitation (CPR) Supplement

WHAT TO DO WHEN THE HEART STOPS

When a casualty's heart stops the First Aider must perform Cardiopulmonary Resuscitation or CPR. CPR is a procedure we use to breath for a casualty and circulate their blood. It is a combination of Rescue Breathing and Chest Compressions (External Cardiac Compressions).

When done correctly this procedure may maintain the casualty's life until more advanced care takes over.

As soon as lack of pulse is evident chest compressions are begun.

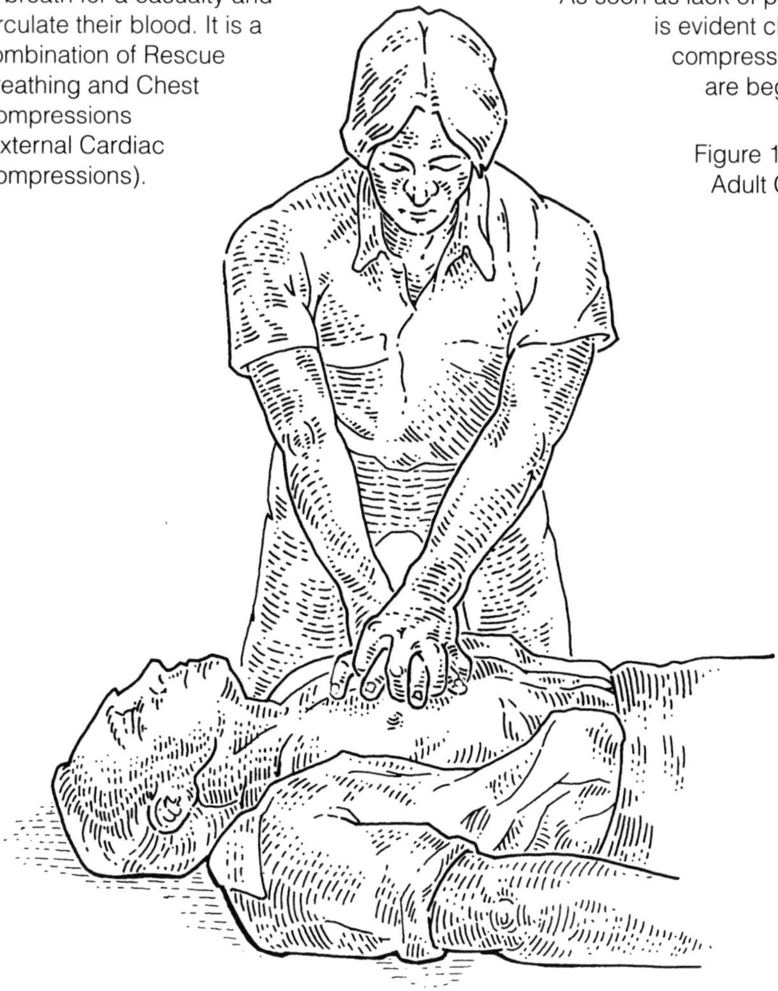

Figure 16.1: Adult CPR

Chest compressions are performed by rhythmically squeezing the heart between the breastbone and the spine. This rhythmic squeezing action causes blood to be circulated.

Alternating this with Rescue Breathing provides oxygen (vital to life) to the bloodstream, to be circulated to the vital organs.

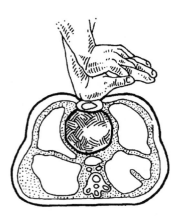

Figure 16.2: The heart as it appears between compressions.

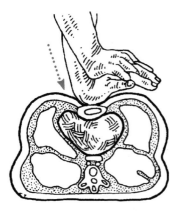

Figure 16.3: The heart, compressed between the breastbone and spine.

Chest Compressions are done by placing the heel of one hand on the chest of the casualty, and laying the other hand on top of the first. The heel of the hand is located directly on the breast bone (sternum) just above the lower tip.

To locate the correct
position for compres-
sions (land–marking) on an
adult and child, slide your fingers
up the casualty's rib–cage with the
hand closest to their feet

Figure 16.4
Feeling the rib–cage

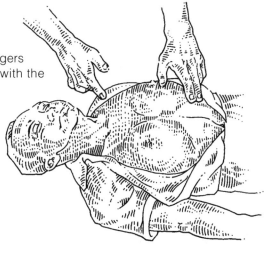

When you reach the point
where the ribs from either side
of the body meet, place your middle
finger in the notch at the base of the
breast bone. Place your index
finger beside the
middle finger.

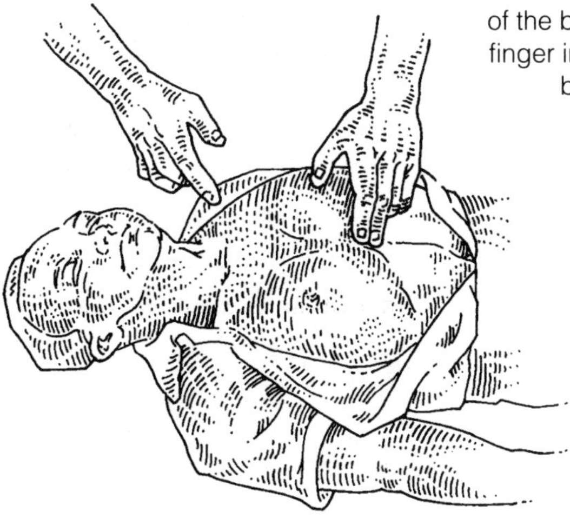

Figure 16.5
Finding the notch

The heel of your other hand is placed along the centre of the breast bone above the index finger.

Locating compressions any lower could cause serious injury and/or ineffective compressions.

Figure 16.6
locating the hand on the chest for CPR

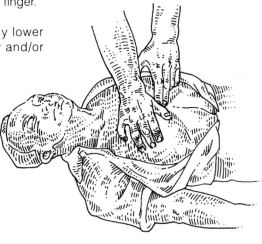

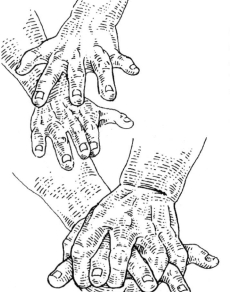

Put the heel of your first hand on top of the hand which is positioned along the breastbone. Interlock your fingers to keep them off the casualty's chest.

Figure 16.7
Hand position for CPR

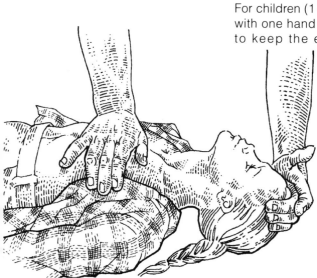

For children (1 – 8 years) compress with one hand only, but remember to keep the elbow locked and shoulders directly over the chest.

Figure 16.8
Child CPR

For infants (under 1 year) the two fingers for administering chest compressions are placed along the breast bone just below an imaginary line drawn between the nipples.

Figure 16.9
Infant CPR
Landmarking

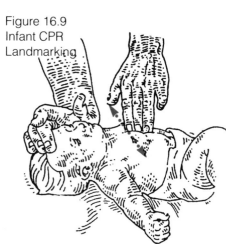

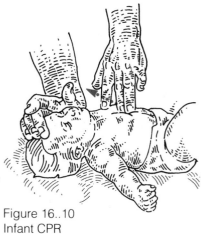

Figure 16..10
Infant CPR
Administering chest compressions

To perform compressions the first aider kneels beside the casualty with their shoulders directly over the casualty's chest. With straight arms and locked elbows the first aider alternately squeezes the chest downward towards the spine and releases upward at the same speed. After performing each set of compressions the first aider ventilates the casualty and then returns to the chest for the next set of compressions.

To perform CPR the casualty must be on a flat surface. Be sure that you have checked pulse for a full 7 seconds (see page 23) prior to beginning CPR. If 'No Pulse' is determined, ensure the EMS has been activated and they know that the casualty has 'No Pulse'. Then find the correct hand position and begin compressions and ventilations.

For Adults

15 compressions (1 1/2 to 2 inches) followed by two slow full breaths (1 to 1 1/2 seconds each). Compress at a rate of 80–100 per minute, or fifteen compressions every 9–11 seconds.

Recheck pulse and breathing after 4 sets of compressions and ventilations.

For Children (1–8 years)

5 compressions (1 to 1 1/2 inches) followed by one full breath (1 to 1 1/2 seconds). Compress at a rate of 80–100 per minute, or five compressions every 3 seconds.

For Infants (birth – 1 year)

5 compressions (1/2 to 1 inch) followed by one small puff of air. Compress at a rate of at least 100 per minute, cr five compressions in less than 3 seconds.

For children and infants, recheck pulse and breathing after 10 sets of compressions and ventilations.

Remember to:

Count out loud, '1 and 2 and 3 and 4 and...' to assist in timing the compressions.

Remember to relocate the correct hand–position every time you return to the chest to perform compressions.

After approximately one minute stop CPR and recheck breathing and pulse — if no help has arrived, now is the time to go for help yourself. If still no pulse and breathing, return to performing CPR.

CPR must be continued until:

1. The casualty's heart and breathing begin again on their own.
2. Another qualified individual takes over.
3. You are too physically exhausted to continue.

Occasionally, ribs crack or break during CPR. If this happens then simply recheck your hand position and continue with CPR.

If the casualty vomits, roll their body to the side as a unit, ensure the vomiting has stopped and the mouth is clear, then roll them back, reassess breathing and pulse, and continue CPR if necessary.

Figure 16.11
Location of the heart and xiphoid process

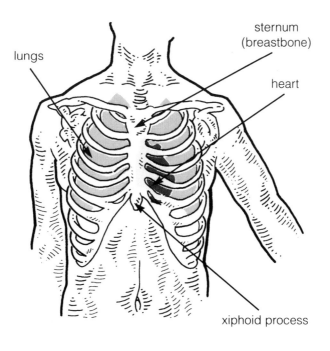

lungs

sternum
(breastbone)

heart

xiphoid process

ONE PERSON CPR – ADULT CASUALTY

STEPS	RESCUE ACTIVITY	MUST DO'S
1	• Establish unresponsiveness • Shout for help • Position the casualty • Open the airway	• Shake casualty's shoulder and ask 'Are you OK?' • Send someone for an ambulance • Turn if necessary • Head tilt / chin lift • If a neck or head injury is suspected, do a jaw thrust (see page 5)
2	• Establish breathlessness • Look, listen and feel for 3 to 5 seconds	• Kneel beside casualty, maintaining open airway • Ear over mouth and nose, observe chest
3	• Breathing —Yes? —No?	• Maintain open airway, proceed to pulse check (see step 5) • Pinch nostrils closed with thumb and forefinger • Seal mouth tightly around casualty's mouth
4	• 2 slow breaths	• Give two slow breaths of air, 1 to 1½ seconds each.
5	• Check pulse • Ensure EMS has been activated	• Maintain head tilt and check the carotid pulse on the side closest to you. (see page 23)
6	• If pulse, continue Rescue Breathing • No pulse, landmark	• One full breath every 5 seconds • Find the correct hand position on the chest
7	• 4 cycles of 15 compressions and 2 ventilations (1 min)	• Proper body position, correct hand position every time, count out loud and ventilate effectively; hand stays on breastbone
8	• Recheck pulse and breathing • If still no pulse or breathing give one breath and repeat step 7.	• Check pulse and breathing for a full 7 seconds • As above, repeat cycles until successful, recheck every few minutes.

ONE PERSON CPR – CHILD CASUALTY

STEPS	RESCUE ACTIVITY	MUST DO'S
1	• Establish unresponsiveness • Shout for help • Position the casualty • Open airway	• Shake casualty's shoulder and ask 'Are you OK?' • Send someone for an ambulance • Turn if necessary • Head tilt / chin lift If a neck or head injury is suspected, do a jaw thrust (see page 5)
2	• Establish breathlessness • Look, listen and feel for 3–5 seconds	• Kneel beside casualty, maintaining open airway • Ear over mouth and nose, observe chest
3	• Breathing—Yes? —No?	• Maintain open airway, proceed to pulse check (see step 5) • Pinch nostrils closed with thumb and forefinger • Seal mouth tightly around casualty's mouth
4	• 2 slow breaths	• Give 2 slow breaths of air, 1 to 1 1/2 seconds each (less force than with an adult)
5	• Check pulse • Ensure EMS has been activated	• Maintain head tilt and check the carotid pulse on the side closest to you (see page 23)
6	• If pulse, continue Rescue Breathing • No pulse, landmark	• One full breath every 4 seconds • Find the correct hand position on the chest
7	• 10 cycles of 5 compres- sions and 1 ventilation (1 min)	• Proper body position, correct hand position every time, count out loud and ventilate effectively; hand stays on breast bone
8	• Recheck pulse and breathing • If still no pulse or breathing give one breath and repeat step 7	• Check pulse and breathing for a full 7 seconds • As above, repeat cycles until suc- cessful, recheck every few minutes

ONE PERSON CPR – INFANT CASUALTY

STEPS	RESCUE ACTIVITY	MUST DO'S
1	• Establish unresponsiveness • Shout for Help • Position the infant • Open the airway • Careful not to overextend the neck	• Tap infant and call their name • Send someone for an ambulance • Turn if necessary • Head tilt / chin lift If a neck or head injury is suspected, gently lift the lower jaw forward without moving the neck Tilt the head only if you cannot inflate the chest (see page 5)
2	• Establish breathlessness • Look, listen and feel for 3 to 5 seconds	• Place your cheek over the infant's mouth and nose • Listen and feel for air, watch for chest movement
3	• Breathing—Yes? • Breathing—No?	• Maintain open airway, proceed to pulse check (see step 5) • Seal your mouth over the infant's mouth and nose
4	• 2 slow puffs	• Give 2 small, slow puffs of air
5	• Check pulse • Ensure EMS has been activated	• Maintain head tilt and check the brachial pulse on the infant (see page 23)
6	• If pulse, continue Rescue Breathing • No pulse; landmark	• One puff every 3 seconds • Find the correct hand postion on the chest
7	• 10 cycles of 5 compressions and 1 ventilation (1 min)	• Proper body position, position finger tips correctly each time, count out loud, ventilate effectively
8	• Recheck pulse and breathing • If still no pulse or breathing give one breath and repeat step 7	• Check pulse and breathing for a full 7 seconds • As above, repeat cycles until successful, recheck every few minutes

Reference: The Journal of the American Medical Association (JAMA), Standards and Guidelines for Cardiopulmonary Resuscitation (CPR) and Emergency Cardiac Care (ECC), June 1986.

APPENDIX

FIRST AID KIT

Contents of a General First Aid Kit

Everyone should have a First Aid kit available at home, in the car or other vehicle, and at recreational and construction sites. You can buy or make a kit. Whichever, it should be compact, efficient and checked regularly to ensure it is clean and complete.

Contents (minimum)

Adhesive tape
Tweezers
Safety Pins
Dressing (gauze)
Triangular Bandages (2)
Adhesive dressing strips (Band-aids)
Pencil and pad
Red Cross First Aid Manual
Emergency telephone numbers
Emergency Blanket
Scissors
Syrup of Ipecac
Change for a phone.

Adhesive Tape

This is available in many forms and widths, and is used to provide pressure, support, or to hold dressings and/or bandages in place. Although very useful to the First Aider it is by no means a necessity.

Gauze

Gauze is the most widely used of all dressings applied directly to open wounds. It is light, cool, loosely woven and absorbent. It comes in various sizes. For a very small wound, use an adhesive strip compress (e.g. bandaid) which is a small pad of gauze on the surface of a strip of adhesive tape. These should be bought in small quantities, since the adhesive spoils with age.

Sterile Dressings

Prepared dressings are sterilized with heat. They are available from a manufacturer in air-tight wrappings to protect them from contamination. At all times First Aiders should exercise great care when opening these packages making sure the surface to be placed on the wound is not contaminated by their hands.

Improvised Dressings

The real test of a First Aider is the ability to **improvise** and make something on the spot. Prepared sterile dressings are not always available. A substitute dressing, such as the inside of a clean, ironed, folded handkerchief, freshly laundered towels, wash cloths or sheets may be necessary. Every effort must be made to not touch the surface to be placed on the wound. If the items mentioned above are not available use clean clothing: a shirt, slip, scarf or blouse.

Container for First Aid Materials

This container should be clean and if possible water proof. Tupperware is a good example of such a container.

Further Acknowledgements

This edition of "First Aid"
was reviewed by:

B. Weitzman, M.D.C.M.,
FRCP(C) CCFP(EM)

Revisions by:

Shelley Shea

Original Design and Layout:

J. Moretta
C.C. Brimley

Illustrations:

J. Gray
A. MacTavish

Index

Abdominal Thrust Technique .... **7 - 10**
Acknowledgements .... **ii, 81**
Airway Management **4**
Alcohol and Drug abuse **34**
Allergic reactions **33**
Animal bites **55**
Artificial respiration .... **14 - 18**
   mouth-to-mouth (or
   mouth to nose, mouth
   to stoma) techniques
Assessments
   initial **2**
   secondary **36**

Back Blows **11, 12, 13**
Back injuries **40, 41**
Bandages **44, 45**
Bee and wasp stings **33, 34**
Bleeding,
   external **20**
   internal **21**
   nosebleed **66**
   scalp and head injuries **38**
   shock **24**
Blood suckers/leeches **56**
Bone and joint injuries **43**
   dislocation **53**
Fractures **43**
   prevention of **43**
   signs and symptoms of **43**
Sprains **52, 53**
Strains **53**
Breathing **14**
   rescue breathing .... **15 - 18**
Burns **59**
   chemical **60**
   electrical **61**
   eye **61**
   First Aid **60, 61**
   prevention of **59**

Cardiopulmonary Resuscitation **81**
Chemical burns **60**
   First Aid
Chest Thrust Technique .... **11 - 13**
Chest wounds **22**

Childbirth **73, 74**
Choking **6**
   First Aid for .... **7 - 13**
   prevention **6**
   signs and symptoms **6**
Circulatory system **19**
Cold exposure .... **62 - 65**
   prevention of **62, 63**
   First Aid **63, 64**
Contact (skin) poisoning **33**
Convulsions **70, 71**
   First Aid for **71**
CPR **81**

Diabetes **71, 72**
Dislocations **53**
Drags and carries .... **76 - 78**
Drugs (and their abuse) **34**

Ear injuries **67**
Emergency medical assistance **35**
Epilepsy **71**
   First Aid
Eye injuries **66**

Face and jaw injuries **44**
Fainting **70**
Fever **72**
First Aid - kits **80**
   legal aspects of .... **iv**
First Aid definition .... **iv**
Food, choking on .... **6 - 13**
Foot and leg injuries .... **50 - 53**
Forearm & wrist fracture **47, 48**
Fractures **43**
   ankle and foot **51, 52**
   collarbone **45, 46**
   compound **43**
   simple **43**
   upper arm **47**
   lower arm **47, 48**
   jaw **44**
   lower leg **51**
   splinting .... **48 - 50**
   upper leg **50**
Frostbite and Frost nip **64, 65**

Index (Cont.)

Head injuries 38
  signs and symptoms
  First Aid
Heart attack 68
  First Aid for 69
  signs and symptoms of 68
Heat exhaustion 61, 62
  First Aid
Heat stroke 62
  First Aid
  signs and symptoms
Hypothermia 63, 64
  First Aid
  prevention of
  signs and symptoms

Identification 37
medical
Impaled objects 22, 23
Infant
  airway management 5
  choking .... 11 - 13
Ingested poisons 27
Initial assessment 2
Insect bites and stings 33, 34, 56
  First Aid
  symptoms

Jaw Thrust Manoeuvre 5
Joint injuries (see Bone and
  joint injuries) 43

Knee 58

Lacerations (see wounds) 54
Lifting .... 75 - 79

Medical identification 37
Mouth-to-mouth (or mouth-to-
  nose) rescue
  breathing 15, 16
  in infants 5, 17, 18
Mouth-to-stoma rescue
  breathing 18

Neck injuries 5, 38
Nose (and nosebleed) 66

Poisons 26
  contact 33
  First Aid 27
  ingested (eaten) 27
  inhaled (breathed) 33
  injected 33, 34
  prevention 26
Pulse check - Adult & Child 23
Pulse check - Infant (Brachial
  Pulse) 23
Pupils 36

Rattlesnakes 57
Rescue breathing 14
Respiratory emergencies (and
  artificial respiration)

Secondary assessment 36
Semi-prone position 25
Shock 24
  signs and symptoms 24
  First Aid 24, 25
Slings .... 44 - 48
Skull fracture 38
Snake-bite 56, 57
  First Aid
  prevention of
  signs and symptoms
Spinal injuries 40
  First Aid 41
  prevention of 41
Splints 48, 49
Sprains 52, 53
  First Aid
  prevention
signs and symptoms
Strains 53
Stretchers 77
Stroke 69
  First Aid
  signs and symptoms
Sucking chest wound 22
Sunburn 61
  First Aid

Index (Cont.)

Ticks.................... **56**
   First Aid for
Transportation............ **75 – 79**
Triangular bandage......... **44, 45**
   application

Unconscious casualty........... **3**

Wounds.................... **54**
   bandaging for.............. **57**
   First Aid.................. **55**
   prevention................. **54**
   signs and symptoms.......... **54**

Addresses of Divisions and National Office

BRITISH COLUMBIA/YUKON
The Canadian Red Cross Society, British Columbia/Yukon Division
4710 Kingsway, Suite 400
Burnaby, B.C. V6H 4M2
(604-431-4200)

ALBERTA/NORTHWEST TERRITORIES
The Canadian Red Cross Society, Alberta/North West Territories Division
737 - 13th Avenue, S.W., Calgary, Alberta T2R 1J1
(403-228-2169)

SASKATCHEWAN
The Canadian Red Cross Society, Saskatchewan Division
2571 Broad Street, Regina, Saskatchewan S4P 3B4
(306-352-4601)

MANITOBA
The Canadian Red Cross Society, Manitoba Division
226 Osborne Street North, Winnipeg, Manitoba R3C 1V4
(204-772-2551)

ONTARIO
The Canadian Red Cross Society, Ontario Division
5700 Cancross Court, Mississauga, Ontario L3R 3E9
(416-890-1000)

QUEBEC
The Canadian Red Cross Society, Quebec Division
2170 René Lévesque Blvd. W., Montreal, Quebec H3H 1R6
(514-937-7761)

NEW BRUNSWICK
The Canadian Red Cross Society, New Brunswick Division
P.O. Box 39, Saint John, N.B. E2L 3X3
(506-648-5000)

PRINCE EDWARD ISLAND
The Canadian Red Cross Society, P.E.I. Division
62 Prince Street, Charlottetown, P.E.I. C1A 4R2
(902-894-8551)

NOVA SCOTIA
The Canadian Red Cross Society, Nova Scotia Division
1940 Gottingen Street, Box 366 Halifax, Nova Scotia B3J 2P8
(902-423-9181)

NEWFOUNDLAND
The Canadian Red Cross Society, Newfoundland Division
7 Wicklow St., St. John's, Newfoundland A1B 4A4
(709-754-0461)

NATIONAL OFFICE
The Canadian Red Cross Society
1800 Alta Vista Drive, Ottawa, Ontario K1G 4J5
(613-739-3000)

List of Figures

FIGURE	TITLE	PAGE
2.1	Obstruction of Airway caused by Tongue	4
2.2	Opened Airway	4
2.3	Jaw Thrust Maneouvre	5
2.4	Jaw Thrust Maneouvre	5
2.5	Choking Distress Signal	6
2.6	Heimlich Manoeuvre (Abdominal Thrusts)	7
2.7	Self Administered Abdominal Thrusts	7
2.8	Heimlich Manoeuvre/Unconscious Casualty	9
2.9, 2.9A	Back Blows for Choking Infant	12
2.10	Chest Thrusts for Choking Infant	12
3.1	Mouth to Mouth Seal - Adult and Child	16
3.2	Mouth to Mouth Technique - Adult and Adult	16
3.3	Mouth to Mouth and Nose Seal - Adult and Infant	16
3.4	Mouth to Nose Technique	18
3.5	Mouth to Stoma Technique	18
4.1	Schematic Circulatory System	19
4.2	Control of Bleeding	20
4.3	First Aid for Severe Bleeding	21
4.4	Schematic: Sucking Chest Wound	22
4.5	First Aid for Impaled Object	23
4.6	Pulse Check (Landmark)	23
4.7	Pulse Check (Location)	23
4.8	Pulse Check (Infant Brachial)	23
5.1	First Aid for Shock	24
5.2	Semi-prone or Recovery Position	25
8.1	Medical Indentification	37
9.1	Immobilization of Head and Neck	38
9.2	Care for Head Injuries	39
9.3	Spinal column/spinal cord	40
9.4	Spinal column/spinal cord damage	42
9.5	Technique for use of spinal board	42
10.1	Major types of fractures	43
10.2	Bandages and knots	45
10.3-10.5	How to Immobilize a Fractured Collarbone	46
10.6-10.7	How to Immobilize an upper arm fracture	47
10.8-10.10	How to Immobilize a lower arm fracture	48

List of Figures (Cont.)

10.11	Types of splints	**49**
10.12-10.15	How to Immobilize an upper leg fracture	**50**
10.16-10.18	How to Immobilize a lower leg fracture	**51**
10.19-10.20	How to Immobilize a fractured foot	**52**
10.21	Immobilizing a fractured ankle	**52**
11.1	Major types of wounds	**54**
11.2	Hand Bandaging	**58**
12.1	Major types of Burns	**60**
14.1	Early Warning signs of Heart Attack	**68**
15.1-15.2	Drag Carry	**75**
15.3	Chair Carry	**76**
15.4-15.5	Hand Seat	**76**
15.6	Human Crutch	**77**
15.7	Improvised Stretchers	**77**
15.8	Blanket Lift	**78**
16.1	Adult CPR	**81**
16.2	Heart between compressions	**82**
16.3	Heart compressed between breastbone and spine . . .	**82**
16.4	Feeling the rib-cage	**83**
16.5	Finding the notch	**83**
16.6	Locating hand on chest for CPR	**84**
16.7	Hand position for CPR	**84**
16.8	Child CPR	**85**
16.9	Infant CPR - landmarking	**85**
16.10	Infant CPR - Administering chest compressions	**85**
16.11	Location of heart and xiphoid process	**87**

List of Tables

FIGURE	TITLE	PAGE
1.1	Initial Assessment Flow Chart	**3**
6.1	Potentially Dangerous Household Poisons	**28**
6.2	Common Poisonous Plants	**30**
8.1	Secondary Assessment	**37**